Trauma and Orthopedic Surgery in Clinical Practice

Paul R. Wood,[†]
Peter F. Mahoney,[‡] **and**
Julian P. Cooper[†]

[†]*University Hospital, Birmingham NHS Foundation Trust*
Birmingham, UK

[‡]*Royal Centre for Defence Medicine, Institute of Research*
and Development, Birmingham, UK

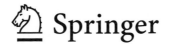 Springer

Paul R. Wood, MB, ChB, FRCA
University Hospital
Birmingham NHS
  Foundation Trust
Birmingham, UK

Peter F. Mahoney, TD, MSc, FRCA,
FFARCSI, FIMC, RCS Edin, DMCC
Royal Centre for Defence Medicine
Institute of Research
  and Development
Birmingham, UK

Julian P. Cooper, MB, ChB, FRCS
University Hospital
Birmingham NHS
  Foundation Trust
Birmingham, UK

ISBN 978-1-84800-338-5   e-ISBN 978-1-84800-339-2
DOI 10.1007/978-1-84800-339-2

British Library Cataloguing in Publication Data
A catalogue record for this book is available from the British Library

Library of Congress Control Number: 2008933288

Printed on acid-free paper

springer.com

Preface

The orthopedic ward can be a challenging location for the recently qualified doctor. The demands and responsibilities in preparing patients for elective orthopedic and acute trauma surgery are often very different. The situation is not helped by the impressive comorbidity often seen in orthopedic patients or the increasing tendency for out-of-hours ward cover to be provided by resident doctors working "off their patch."

In this book, the authors have attempted to provide a practical guide to the most common perioperative issues and medical problems found during the day-to-day management of these patients.

The model used is based on an earlier "in-house" publication written for the guidance of anesthetic trainees working in a trauma intensive care unit. The authors are all hardened observers of the speed at which today's recommendations become yesterday's history and so have made a particular effort to select references that will assist in readers remaining updated.

Contents

Preface.   v

Notes for the Reader.   xi

Section 1:   The Orthopedic Ward, Orthopedic Patients,
             and Procedures

1   Patients and Procedures.   3
    Part I   3
    Part II.   3
    Orthopedic Glossary.   3
    Radiology.   3

2   The Ward Team.   21

3   The Ward Round.   23

Section 2:   Patient Management

4   Preparing Patients for Operation.   29
    Part I: Medical Preparation   29
    Part II: Consent and Identification   52

5   Intravenous Fluids and Electrolytes   57
    Fluids Used in Routine Practice.   57
    Fluid Management: Some Practical Observations   60
    Sodium and Potassium Disturbances
    on the Orthopedic Ward.   63

6   Analgesia   65
    Assessment of Pain   65
    Methods of Treating Pain   66
    Problems Associated With Analgesia.   68

7   Dressings, Drains, Plasters, and Tubes   71

Section 3:   Special Patient Groups

8   The Patient With a Fractured Neck of Femur   79
     Surgical Classification of Proximal
     Femur Fractures   79
     Principles of Management   81
     Your Responsibilities   83

9   Rheumatoid Arthritis   87
     General Considerations   87
     Preparation For Surgery   87
     Postoperative Care   88

10   Hemophilia   89
     Background   89
     Orthopedic Presentation   89
     Preoperative Preparation   90
     Postoperative Care   90

Section 4:   Problems and Complications: The Patient

11   Infection and Immunocompromise   95
     Definitions   95
     Vulnerability to Infection   95
     History and Examination   96
     Laboratory and Radiological Investigation
     of Infection   96
     Postoperative Infection   96
     Principles of Managing Infected
     or Immunocompromised Patients   99
     The Risk to Yourself   101

12   Compartment Syndrome   103
     The Problem   103
     Causes   103
     Prevention   104
     Recognition   104
     Treatment   105

13   Deep Venous Thrombosis and
     Pulmonary Embolism   109
     Deep Venous Thrombosis   109
     Pulmonary Embolus   110

14   Fat Embolism   113
     Presentation   113

Confirming the Diagnosis.   114
Treatment   114

15 The Confused Patient   115
Precipitating Factors.   115
The Alcoholic Patient   116
Risks of Confusion   116
Principles of Management of Confusion   116

16 The Ill Patient and Medical Emergencies   119
Principles of Management   119
Medical Emergencies   123

17 Problems With Blood Transfusion.   131
Pretransfusion.   132
Transfusion   133
Posttransfusion   133
Responding to a Transfusion Problem.   133

Section 5:   Problems and Complications: The Doctor

18 Medical Errors   137
Background.   137
Causes of Medical Error and Avoiding Them   137
What to Do If You Have Made a Mistake   138

Section 6:   When Treatment Stops

19 Do Not Resuscitate Orders, Death Certification,
and the Coroner   143
When Further Treatment Is Thought
Inappropriate   143
Do Not Resuscitate Orders.   143
Certification of Death   144
Cremation Certificates   144
Postmortems   144
Reporting to the Coroner   144

Bibliography and Further Reading   147

Index   149

Notes for the Reader

The authors have written this book mindful of the fact that undergraduate medical education continues to evolve. Qualification produces graduates who are comfortable with the science, philosophy, and ethics of medicine, but the practical know-how required to manage patients is still largely acquired in a piecemeal fashion while carrying out daily duties.

This is not a textbook; it is intended as a practical working manual to guide you on the adult orthopedic ward. The book begins with an overview of orthopedic procedures and patients. Thereafter, it is split into sections that approximate the pre-, peri-, and postoperative phases.

Each subject discussion ends with suggested further reading that directs you to other parts of the book that contain supporting material.

It is intended to help you spot potential problems and thus avoid them.

When difficulties or complications occur, it offers practical advice based on safe principles of acute care. It is no substitute for experience, which is why you will repeatedly see phrases that convey the same message, which is "get help." We make no apology for such repetition.

Current medical knowledge is constantly being revised, and access to such information is increasingly disseminated by electronic means; consequently, external references are listed at the end of the book, including Web sites to review the latest developments as necessary.

We do not discuss the specialist areas of pediatrics, spinal surgery, or orthopedic surgical oncology. The management of the multiply injured patient is also missing; such patients have no place on the general orthopedic ward.

Finally, we do not know it all and consequently will be grateful for readers' comments.

Section I
The Orthopedic Ward, Orthopedic Patients, and Procedures

Chapter 1
Patients and Procedures

PART I

Table 1.1 provides an overview of the various conditions associated with elective or emergency admissions to a general adult orthopedic ward.

FURTHER READING

See Patients and Procedures: Part II and Orthopedic Glossary in this chapter.

PART II

Table 1.2 provides more details on some of the techniques listed in Part I of this chapter and provide notes regarding patients.

FURTHER READING

See Patients and Procedures: Part I and Orthopedic Glossary in this chapter.

ORTHOPEDIC GLOSSARY

Table 1.3 provides a minidictionary of terms concerning orthopedic methods and hardware that you may hear or see on ward rounds and in patients' notes. They may assist in writing operating lists, understanding operation notes, and in comprehending some of your orthopedic seniors more esoteric discussions.

FURTHER READING

See Patients and Procedures: Parts I and II in this chapter.

RADIOLOGY

Imaging studies have had a fundamental role in orthopedics ever since the discovery of X-rays. Other imaging methods also have application in orthopedic and trauma management; selection of

P. Wood et al., *Trauma and Orthopedic Surgery in Clinical Practice*,
DOI: 10.1007/978-1-84800-339-2_1, © Springer-Verlag London Limited 2009

TABLE 1.1. Orthopedic Pathology

	Elective	Emergency
BONES	**Postfracture:** 1. Healed injury: Removal of metal work 2. Nonunion, delayed union, and malunion: May be complex, possibly involving removal of metal work, bone grafting, osteotomy, refixation **Infection:** 1. Drainage and bony debridement 2. Bone transport or other ring fixator technique **Tumor:** 1. Biopsy 2. Curettage/excision (for benign lesions) 3. Prophylactic fixation: For impending pathological fracture 4. Endoprosthesis (excision and massive replacement of bone) 5. Amputation **Deformity:** 1. Limb lengthening: Usually with ring fixator 2. Correction of deformity: By osteotomy or gradual correction with ring fixator	**Fractures** are treated by reduction and then stabilization: *Reduction:* 1. Closed: Fracture not directly seen, usually monitored by X-ray 2. Open: Fracture ends seen in the wound and brought into a satisfactory position *Stabilization:* 1. Closed: Fracture held by cast, traction, bracing 2. Minimally invasive: Fracture not opened and implants usually inserted out of zone of injury (e.g., K-wires, external fixation, intramedullary nail and some plates) 3. Open: Plates and screws **Infection:** 1. Biopsy: To obtain diagnostic material for culture 2. Drainage

JOINTS	**Degenerative change:**	**Dislocations** require urgent reduction:
	1. Soft tissue procedures (e.g., arthroscopic debridement)	1. Closed: Most common
	2. Osteotomy: Realignment of a joint by cutting a bone adjacent to it	2. Open
	3. Fusion: Surgical abolition of joint and all movement	Occasionally, fracture fixation or acute ligament repairs are needed to maintain joint stability.
	4. Arthroplasty: Includes joint replacement and joint excision (Girdlestone)	**Infection** of a joint, septic arthritis, requires urgent diagnosis and treatment:
	Others:	1. Aspiration: To obtain diagnostic material for culture
	1. Soft tissue reconstruction for instability (e.g., anterior cruciate ligament reconstruction)	2. Joint washout:
	2. Procedures for impingement (e.g., subacromial decompression in the shoulder)	a. Arthroscopic
	3. Removal of loose bodies: Usually arthroscopic	b. Open, via formal arthrotomy
		3. Open joint debridement
SOFT TISSUES[a]	**Tendon and muscle:**	**Trauma:**
	1. Reconstruction of chronically damaged tendons (e.g., rotator cuff repair)	1. Debridement of devitalized tissues
	2. Treatments for abnormal tendons (e.g., tennis elbow release, Achilles tendon decompression)	2. Tendon, vessel, and nerve repair
	3. Release of chronic compartment syndrome	3. Fasciotomy for acute compartment syndrome
	4. Tendon transfers (e.g., to compensate for radial nerve palsy)	4. Wound closure: The reconstructive ladder:
	Nerve:	a. Direct wound closure (immediate or delayed)
	1. Release of nerve compression (e.g., carpal tunnel decompression)	b. Skin graft[a]
	2. Grafting of chronically damaged nerves	i. Split skin
		ii. Full thickness
		c. Flap cover[a]
		i. Local
		ii. Distant (pedicle or free transfer)

[a]These procedures are usually undertaken with plastic surgeons.

TABLE 1.2. Orthopedic Techniques

Procedure	Principle	Patient Comments
1. Closed reduction of fractures and dislocations	Bones and joints returned to satisfactory alignment. Sufficient stability for position to be maintained with external or no splintage.	Plasters and other splints may cause limb compression; careful assessment of compartments and neurovascular status required afterward.
2. Traction	Maintains limb alignment and counteracts shortening from muscle spasm. Holds fracture in safe position before definitive treatment.	Not ordinarily used for long periods in modern trauma practice owing to hazards of prolonged immobilization and effective operative methods
3. External fixation (ex-fix)	External "scaffolding" joined to bone by pins crossing the skin. Rapidly stabilizes bones and soft tissues as a temporary measure (e.g., while swelling resolves) and less commonly as definitive treatment of a fracture. Some specialized techniques are used to lengthen bone and correct deformity.	Used in the initial management of complicated limb trauma with open fractures. Wound closure is often delayed, and infection is a constant risk.
4. Percutaneous pinning (K-wires)	Small bones (e.g., in the hand) held in position by smooth, thin pins inserted across the fracture, usually though the skin.	Wires may irritate soft tissues and increase the risk of infection. They may loosen and be dislodged or even break. If severe swelling occurs, wires might disappear beneath the skin.

5. Rigid internal fixation	Bony anatomical relationships maintained in a rigid fashion usually by plates and screws, while healing occurs. Often used for injuries in or near joints (e.g., sliding hip screw for extracapsular hip fractures, cannulated screws for intracapsular fractures).	Most fixation of this type requires open procedures that directly expose the fracture site. This may compromise local blood supply and increase the risk of problems with bone healing and infection. There is a risk of injury to vessels and nerves traversing the operative area. Prominence of plates or other symptoms may mandate removal of the metal work later. Compartments must be monitored carefully. Operations for fractured neck of femur and other common fractures in the elderly require careful preparation owing to the frequency and severity of comorbidities.
6. Intramedullary nails	The nail is inserted into the marrow cavity of long bones after reaming to size. Stability is enhanced by locking screws inserted through the nail at both ends. In modern practice, the fracture site is rarely opened, preserving local periosteal blood supply.	Reaming of the marrow cavity may produce fat emboli, causing postoperative respiratory problems. As with any procedure involving insertion of metal implants, there is a risk of infection. Compartments must be monitored carefully.

(Continued)

TABLE 1.2. (Continued)

Procedure	Principle	Patient Comments
7. Joint replacement (replacement arthroplasty)	Total and unicompartmental joint replacement is done electively to treat osteoarthritis and other destructive joint conditions (e.g., avascular necrosis of the femoral head). Replacement of one side of the joint only (hemiarthroplasty) is almost always performed following fractures that have an unacceptable risk of failure if internally fixed (e.g., displaced intracapsular fractured neck of femur in frail elderly patients).	Elective cases; patients are often obese. Prophylaxis against venous thromboembolism is necessary. Postop analgesia can be difficult. Increasingly, patients who have outlived their prosthesis require revision of their original arthroplasty, perhaps 20 years or more after the original procedure. These revisions are often prolonged and involve substantial blood loss, and postop analgesia can cause problems. Infection in a joint replacement is a disaster: Bacteremia must be avoided (e.g., gentamicin cover for urethral catheterization postoperatively). Hemiarthroplasty for fractures in frail patients: Same as for Procedure 5. Some patients will sustain periprosthetic fractures (e.g., at the tip of a hip replacement), usually requiring complex, lengthy intervention.

| 8. Arthroscopy | Telescopic examination of the inside of a joint. Insertion of additional instruments allows diagnosis and treatment of joint pathology. In today's practice, most arthroscopy is therapeutic, rather than purely diagnostic, with the pathology having been identified by magnetic resonance imaging (MRI) scanning.

Very common procedure. Most joints can be arthroscoped, but the knee and shoulder are most common. | Frequently younger day case patients, often following sporting injury.
Postop pain (especially shoulders) caused by the joint being distracted with irrigating fluid plus the use of bone sutures can be an issue. Infection is also a risk. |

TABLE 1.3. Common Orthopedic Terms

AO (*Arbeitsgemeinschaft für Osteosynthesefragen*)	The initials (in German) of an organization devoted to the study of methods of fixation of fractures, originally founded in Switzerland in 1958. The AO "brand" is applied to specific implant designs, a fracture classification system, and educational courses.
Ankylosis	Spontaneous bony fusion of a joint as part of a pathological process.
Antegrade	A direction in a bone from proximal to distal, typically used to describe the direction of insertion of intramedullary nails (cf. *retrograde*).
Arthrodesis	Surgical bony fusion of a joint; usually performed for osteoarthritis.
Arthroplasty	A surgical procedure on a joint that aims to restore function. Although this is usually used to refer to joint replacement surgery, other procedures fall into this category, notably *excision* arthroplasty—the surgical removal of a joint (see *Girdlestone*).
ASIF (Association for the Study of Internal Fixation)	The English translation of *AO* (see *AO* entry), mainly used in North America.
Cancellous screw	A screw designed for placement in cancellous bone (typically found in the *metaphysis* and *epiphysis*).
Cannulated screw	A hollow screw inserted over a guidewire previously inserted across a fracture. Ensures that the final position of the screw is known prior to insertion. Most commonly used to fix certain intracapsular fractured necks of femur.
Cement	Acrylic bone cement used to support certain joint replacements by filling the space between the prosthesis and the bone. The cement thus placed is often termed the cement *mantle*.
Cortical screw	A screw designed for fixation in hard cortical bone (typically found in the *diaphysis*). Often used in other areas as well.
Countersink	A tool used to create a recess in the surface of a bone to accept the head of a screw. This optimizes force transmission to the bone, prevents loss of compression, and reduces prominence of the screw (important in areas such as joints).

DCP (dynamic compression plate)	A type of metal plate used to fix fractures. The design of holes in the plate allows the fracture fragments to be compressed together by appropriate screw insertion.
Delayed union	A complication of fracture healing in which the fracture fails to heal within the expected time frame (cf. *nonunion*).
Denham pin	A type of *skeletal traction* pin characterized by a short thread in the middle that is designed to sit in the bone and prevent the pin from slipping sideways (cf. *Steinmann pin*).
Diaphysis (adjective: diaphyseal)	The shaft part of a long bone. It typically has a thick cortex of compact bone and an essentially hollow medulla (marrow cavity).
Dynamic hip screw (DHS)	A commercial make of screw and plate used to fix certain types of hip fracture (see *Sliding hip screw* and Fig. 8.5.
Dynamization	A procedure designed to allow the ends of a fixed fracture either to come together or to move in a controlled fashion (or both). This is generally done with the object of promoting healing when healing seems slow. In a nailed fracture, this involves removal of one or more locking screws from one end of the nail.
Epiphysis (adjective: epiphyseal)	One of the ends of a bone, often part of a joint with another bone.
Exchange nailing	A procedure usually designed to promote fracture healing and occasionally to treat infection after a nailed fracture. In essence, the original nail is removed and replaced with a new, thicker nail, after *reaming* of the medullary canal.
External fixation	A method of bone stabilization characterized by an external framework connected to the bone by pins that cross the skin.
Girdlestone procedure	An excision *arthroplasty* of the hip joint. In the past, this was performed for tuberculous infection or painful osteoarthritis of the hip but now is generally reserved for complications of joint replacement (e.g., intractable infection.)
Grub screw	A headless screw used to prevent loosening of other components.

(Continued)

TABLE 1.3. (Continued)

Hemiarthroplasty	A joint replacement that replaces one half of the joint only, most commonly the hip and shoulder after fractures. Examples include Thompson (Figure 8.3) and Austin Moore hemiarthroplasties, which replace the head of the femur in the fractured neck of femur.
Hoffman	A commercial make of external fixation system used to treat fractures.
Ilizarov (frame)	A particular type of external fixation in which bone is connected to a circular frame, often by way of highly tensioned fine wires. The system is useful for correction of deformity, lengthening bones, and treatment of very complex fractures, especially where there is infection or bone loss.
Instability (fracture)	The tendency of a fracture to lose position when exposed to physiological loading before healing occurs. Loosely speaking, instability is how "wobbly" the fracture is.
Instability (joint)	Symptomatic, unwanted movement of a joint.
Internal fixation	A method of bone stabilization by which the (usually metal) implants are entirely within the soft tissue envelope. Essentially refers to plates, screws, nails, and certain types of bone wiring.
Intramedullary nail (or rod)	A method of bone stabilization by which a metal rod is inserted across the fracture within the marrow cavity (*medullary canal*) of the bone. Modern nails are secured at each end with *locking screws*, which greatly increase the range of fractures that can be managed by nailing.
Kirschner (K-) wires	Sharp pointed thin wires used percutaneously or at open operation to maintain reduction of fractures, often as a temporary fixation during the operation itself but also as definitive fixation.
Lag screw	A bone screw inserted across a fracture in such a way that compression is generated between the fracture ends.
LCP (locking compression plate)	A commercial example of *locking plate* that also allows screws to be used in the more conventional manner as in the *DCP*.

LISS (less-invasive stabilization system) plate	A commercial *locking plate* used for *MIPPO* fixation of distal femoral and proximal tibial fractures.
Locking plate	A design of bone plate in which the screws fix rigidly not only to the bone but also to the plate. Such a plate is mechanically equivalent to an external fixator but lies within the soft tissue envelope. Sometimes confusingly termed an *internal fixator*.
Locking screws	1. Screws inserted at the proximal and distal ends (one or both) of an *intramedullary nail* to prevent rotation and maintain length of a bone.
	2. Strictly speaking, locking *head* screws. Special screws designed to screw into bone and into a *locking plate*.
Malunion	The healing of a fracture in an unacceptable position.
Metaphysis (adjective: metaphyseal)	The parts of a long bone where the shaft becomes wider toward the ends.
MIPPO or MIPO	Acronym for **m**inimally invasive **p**ercutaneous **p**late **o**steosynthesis. The first "P" is often dropped. A technique for fracture plating in which the plate and screws are introduced through small incisions, thereby reducing the surgical trauma to the fracture site.
Nail	See *Intramedullary nail*.
Nonunion	A complication of a fracture in which healing ceases or cannot complete.
ORIF (open reduction and internal fixation)	An operative procedure for fracture stabilization in which the fracture reduction is achieved under direct vision and secured (usually) with screws or plates.
Osteotomy	An operative procedure that involves cutting a bone. Typical applications are to correct malunion of a fracture or to realign a joint to improve mechanics in osteoarthritis.
Physis (adjective: physeal)	The growth plate in a growing bone; a bone may have several in the growing skeleton, each of which fuses at skeletal maturity, leaving a white line (*physeal scar*) visible on X-ray images.

(Continued)

TABLE 1.3. (Continued)

Procurvatum	Descriptive term for a deformity in which the part in question is bowed convex anteriorly. The opposite of *recurvatum*.
Pseudarthrosis	The development of an abnormal synovial joint between two bones or two fracture fragments, usually as a result of nonunion between the fragments.
Reaming	Preparation of a long bone medullary canal to accept an appropriate size orthopedic implant (e.g., a joint replacement or intramedullary nail).
Recon (reconstruction) plate	A bone fixation plate that can be contoured from side to side as well as top to bottom (as in the *DCP*). This allows it to be used on bones with complex shapes such as the pelvis or distal humerus.
Recurvatum	Descriptive term for a deformity in which the part in question is bowed convex posteriorly. The opposite of *procurvatum*.
Retrograde	A direction in a bone from distal to proximal, typically used to describe the direction of insertion of intramedullary nails (the opposite of *antegrade*). Mainly refers to certain types of femoral and humeral nails.
Self-tapping	A type of bone screw that cuts its own complementary thread as it is inserted. Conventional bone screws usually require the use of a tap to create a thread for the screw in the bone.
Skeletal traction	Application of traction to a fracture or joint via a metal pin inserted across a bone.
Sliding hip screw	A fixed angle screw and plate fixation device usually used to fix extracapsular hip fractures, although certain intracapsular fractures are also suitable. The screw can slide within the plate when the patient bears weight, improving fracture compression.
Steinmann pin	A type of *skeletal traction* pin that is smooth along its length (cf. *Denham pin*).

Tension band principle

A biomechanical principle utilized in fracture fixation by application of a fixation device that converts distracting forces into compression across the fracture. This may be achieved by most types of fixation device but is commonly achieved with a wire configuration in the olecranon or patella—hence "tension band *wiring*" of these fractures.

Valgus

Descriptive term for a deformity in which the part distal to the part in question is directed away from the midline (e.g., valgus knees = knock-kneed). Implicit in this definition is that the part proximal to the deformity must be "placed" (mentally) in its anatomical position.

Varus

Descriptive term for a deformity in which the part distal to the part in question is directed toward the midline (e.g., varus knees = bowlegged). See the caveat under *valgus*.

the appropriate method is an important skill. In this section, the choice of imaging is discussed.

TABLE 1.4. Imaging Modalities

Modality	Orthopedic Uses	Special Points
Plain films[a] Increasingly acquired and displayed digitally. Familiarity with the functions of your picture archiving and communications system (PACS) system is vital.	1. Screening: Chest and pelvic films for injury and hemorrhage in polytrauma 2. Diagnosis: a. Fractures	Obtained in the primary survey of trauma resuscitation Two views at right angles; for shaft fractures, the joint above and below should be shown.
	b. Joint conditions	Most types of arthritis have characteristic X-ray changes.
	c. Bone tumors and infection	Other modalities, especially MRI and nuclear medicine, are often required to refine the diagnosis.
	3. Preoperative planning and preparation	Anesthetic related (e.g., chest X-ray, cervical spine in rheumatoid arthritis) Surgery related: films required for selection of surgical strategy and certain cases require templating to choose the correct implant
	4. Postoperative documentation	A check X-ray may be required if there is inadequate intraoperative imaging. The surgeon's postoperative instructions or protocol will usually make this clear.

(Continued)

TABLE 1.4. (Continued)

Modality	Orthopedic Uses	Special Points
	5. Monitoring	The healing of a fracture or development of a condition such as osteoarthritis or loosening after joint replacement can be monitored using plain films.
Fluoroscopy[a] Intraoperative imaging using an image intensifier (uses low-dose X-rays to provide an immediate television picture of the bone).	1. Guidance for insertion of orthopedic implants, especially in fracture surgery 2. Confirmation of site of surgery (usually in the spine) or injection	It is usually necessary to warn the X-ray department regarding which cases may require a radiographer to operate the image intensifier.
Computed tomography (CT)[a] X-ray-based technique that provides extremely good information about bone. It is also able to demonstrate soft tissues far better than plain films.	1. Polytrauma: Diagnosis of life-threatening head, chest, and abdominal injuries. Increasingly used as default imaging technique for the cervical spine. 2. Diagnosis and preoperative planning for complex fractures (e.g., pelvic and acetabular fractures) 3. Guided drainage and biopsy (e.g., of psoas abscess)	As a technique, is used far less in elective orthopedics than in trauma applications.
Magnetic resonance imaging (MRI) Provides unrivaled depiction of soft tissue anatomy and pathology	1. Demonstration of soft tissue abnormalities (e.g., meniscal tears in the knee, rotator cuff tears in the shoulder, disc prolapse in the spine)	Care must be taken in patients with certain metal implants or foreign bodies. Ferromagnetic objects may migrate with dangerous consequences or if

2. Diagnosis and staging of soft tissue and bone tumors
3. Diagnosis and monitoring of musculoskeletal infection

near the area of interest may cause significant artifact.

Ultrasound

May have advantages over MRI, especially if a dynamic examination is required (e.g., the probe can be moved to examine a tender area)

1. Demonstration of soft tissue abnormalities, especially tendon and ligament abnormalities
2. Detection of foreign bodies
3. Guided injection, aspiration, and biopsy of suspicious areas

Ultrasound is an operator-dependent examination. Musculoskeletal ultrasound requires great skill and experience.

Nuclear medicine[a]

In orthopedics, mainly confined to isotope bone scanning, which reflects blood flow to bone

1. Detection of skeletal metastases
2. Diagnosis and monitoring of infection
3. Diagnosis of occult fractures

It is important to be clear about the clinical question, for example, is the area of interest the whole body, as when looking for metastases, or a single area, as when looking for an occult fracture (e.g., scaphoid).

Some neoplastic conditions (e.g., myeloma) may give negative bone scans. Other techniques such as CT and MRI are supplanting isotope techniques for fracture diagnosis.

---

[a]These techniques require the use of ionizing radiation, requiring special consideration in women of child-bearing age.

Selection of appropriate imaging techniques can be difficult (Table 1.4). It is important to state the clinical question clearly on the request form. This will allow the imaging team to check whether another investigation might give more information and help the radiologist reporting the investigation to provide a definitive answer. In some cases, discussing the problem directly with the radiologist is the most productive way forward; by asking "How can you show me whether the femoral head is invaded with metastasis?" rather than saying "I want a CT of the hip," one might actually find a different investigation is most appropriate.

Chapter 2
The Ward Team

You will quickly discover that the spectrum of age and disease processes outlined in the introductory section on patients and procedures means that the care of these patients is truly multi-disciplinary. Your working day will be made much easier if you strive to establish a working relationship with the various professional groups represented. This is particularly important as (in the United Kingdom at least) you no longer benefit from certain key advantages that did exist by belonging to a traditional surgical firm headed by the consultant in charge.

It is invidious to select any one group for special mention as the process of optimizing and speeding up the whole process of patient admission to discharge is a cooperative effort.

The role of the physiotherapist is fundamental in postoperative progress, and any concerns raised by the physiotherapist merit your undivided attention. Physicians with an interest in the care of the elderly are not universal on orthopedic wards, but there is good evidence that when present their contribution can transform the perioperative care of patients. If such an individual works on your ward, take every opportunity to advance your knowledge of general medicine.

Another group with increasing influence are the intensive care outreach team. These nurses and doctors from the intensive care unit (ICU) will monitor patients recently discharged from ICU to the ward and will also act to provide surveillance and practical hands-on assistance for seriously ill patients.

Certain orthopedic patients will present frustrating problems with pain control. Your key allies here are the nurses and anesthetists who regularly visit as the acute pain control team. They will monitor any specialized form of postoperative analgesia and assist in the management of concurrent medication and postoperative nausea and vomiting.

Your prescribing in general (and mistakes in particular) is unlikely to miss the radar of the pharmacists, who will regularly

P. Wood et al., *Trauma and Orthopedic Surgery in Clinical Practice*,
DOI: 10.1007/978-1-84800-339-2_2, © Springer-Verlag London Limited 2009

review and annotate handwritten prescription charts. Many a serious error has been avoided by their supervision.

The nursing profession contains a plethora of specialists. Respect their particular expertise and be guided by their experience.

Finally, never minimize the contributions made by the auxiliary nursing staff, phlebotomists, ward clerks, domestics, porters, and pastoral caregivers.

Chapter 3
The Ward Round

As an orthopedic junior doctor, one of your prime duties is to see the patients on the ward on a regular basis. After the initial perioperative period or recovery from a fracture, it is likely that little will change day to day in the medical condition of your patients, but it is essential that each patient is seen by a doctor from the team daily to ensure that important problems are not missed. This is particularly the case in elderly patients after fractured neck of femur and similar injuries.

In practice, ward rounds come in several varieties of varying purpose and formality. Table 3.1 indicates the type, purposes, and priorities of the rounds. If possible, a member of nursing staff should be present on the more formal rounds; this might not always be possible at busy times. Physiotherapists are also very helpful to have on ward rounds. Whatever the type of round, it is essential that any changes in a patient's medical care are passed on to the nursing staff, either directly or immediately after the round.

It is of paramount importance that each visit to the patient is recorded in the notes. The entry should indicate who saw the patient, what was found, what was done, and in the case of important information about results, complications, or prognosis, what was said to the patient. Each entry must be signed, legible, dated, and timed.

P. Wood et al., *Trauma and Orthopedic Surgery in Clinical Practice*,
DOI: 10.1007/978-1-84800-339-2_3, © Springer-Verlag London Limited 2009

TABLE 3.1. Description of Rounds

Type	Purposes	Priorities

Informal patient review
Usually junior doctor alone
	Ensuring basic medical care occurs	Checking medical condition:
		  Observations
		  Pain
		  Chest
		  Evidence of venous thromboembolism
		  Surgical wound
		  Drains and catheters
		Housekeeping tasks (checking prescriptions, writing up fluids, cannulas, etc.)

Daily "business" round Junior doctor with middle-grade doctors	Setting priorities for the day Identifying changes from previous day Keeping medical, nursing, and therapy teams informed	Checking medical condition (as above) Housekeeping tasks (as above)

Preoperative round
Junior doctor with operating surgeon
	Ensuring proper preparation for surgery	Checking:
		  Fitness
		  Consent
		  Marking of site
		  Availability of investigation results

Postoperative round
Junior doctor with operating surgeon
	Ensuring appropriate recovery and outcome from surgery	Checking:
		  Pain
		  Junior doctor with operating surgeon
		  Limb neurological function and vascularity
		  Compartments
		  Dressings and casts (to ensure not too tight and no oozing through)
		  Observations
		  Urine output

Postcall ward round Admitting consultant and team	Review of new emergency patients and decision making about management	Check medical condition Ensure availability of important results on which decisions will be made Record keeping especially important

(Continued)

TABLE 3.1. (Continued)

Type	Purposes	Priorities
Consultant ward round The whole surgical team	Formal review of situation and progress Decisions and explanations about strategy Communication of results of surgery and prognosis	Check medical condition Ensure availability of relevant results Record keeping especially important

FURTHER READING

See Patients and procedures Parts I and II in this chapter; Part I, Medical Preparation, and Part II, Consent and Identification, in Chapter 4, Preparing Patients for Operation; and Sections 5 and 6, Problems and Complications.

Section 2
Patient Management

Chapter 4
Preparing Patients for Operation

PART I: MEDICAL PREPARATION

History, Physical Examination, and Clinical Investigations

Introduction
The medical preparation of a patient for a surgical procedure is a two-stage process of identifying actual or potential medical comorbidity and if necessary improving it. The second part assumes that not only is improvement possible, but also it is achievable. While there may not be time in a limb- or life-threatening emergency, it may be necessary before elective surgery (Figure 4.1).

After taking a history and performing a physical examination, two fundamental questions often arise:

1. What is the potential impact of this patient's history and physiological condition on their subsequent anesthesia, surgery, and postoperative recovery.
2. What further tests or investigations (if any) are required? This apparently straightforward question can cause unnecessary delay and cancellations to subsequent surgery if unasked

Two key principles apply:

1. The purpose of any investigation is to further identify or quantify physiological abnormality for which medical intervention prior to surgery will benefit the patient.
2. As a corollary, tests that are unlikely to assist in this aim are usually unwarranted.

Identifying Problems Early: The Preoperative Assessment Clinic
Outpatient assessment before elective surgery allows identification of morbidity and provides the opportunity for improvement before hospital admission. In these clinics, patients are often

P. Wood et al., *Trauma and Orthopedic Surgery in Clinical Practice,*
DOI: 10.1007/978-1-84800-339-2_4, © Springer-Verlag London Limited 2009

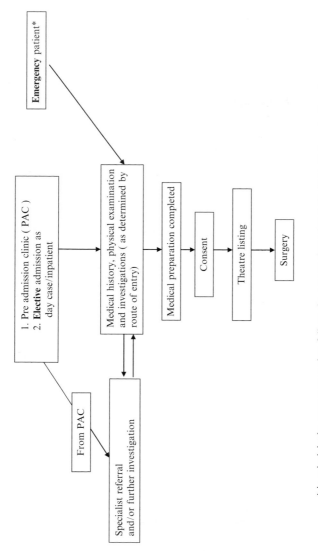

* in principle the emergency patient follows the same pathway but their diagnosis may significantly reduce the time available for preoperative preparation

FIGURE 4.1. The surgical pathway: Admission to operation.

screened first by nurses, and you may then be asked to "preclerk" the patient prior to subsequent admission. This arrangement affords several advantages:

1. Suitably fit patients (selected on the basis of physiological function) can be assigned as day cases.
2. Both known and unsuspected morbidity can be identified and assessed.
3. Patient education can be provided in respect to general risk factors (smoking and obesity) and current medication.
4. The need to obtain old notes because of previous anesthetic or surgical complications or because some specific details of a previous operation (e.g., type of metalwork inserted) is identified.
5. The patient can undergo routine investigations (described here) on the same visit.
6. Most important, the patient can be discussed with or referred to other specialists as necessary before giving the patient a definitive date for an operation.

The same process occurs with elective inpatients who have bypassed the preadmission clinic or emergency admissions; in these situations, unforeseen cancellation or delay of surgery becomes more likely.

Problems Identified During the History and Physical Examination

Heart Disease

1. Ischemic heart disease is common. Routine inquiry about the frequency of recent angina attacks and the response to the patient's usual treatment must be backed up with a 12-lead electrocardiogram (ECG). Patients who have sustained a recent (≤6 weeks) documented myocardial infarction or those complaining of increasing frequency/severity of chest pain are a special risk group and will require cardiology assessment prior to elective surgery.
2. Cardiac failure is also not unusual. The clinical history and examination should establish that this is well controlled. If not, the patient must be referred for further medical management as he or she otherwise presents an unacceptable operative risk.
3. A history or finding of an arrhythmia requires an ECG (unless the problem is obviously benign), and some patients may warrant a period of continuous bedside monitoring (i.e., if the problem is intermittent and the diagnosis uncertain). Atrial fibrillation is a common problem in the elderly, and a rapid

uncontrolled rate needs correction prior to any nonemergency surgery.

4. Patients with valvular abnormalities are frequently aware that they "have a murmur," and their old medical notes may document the cause and subsequent management. Beware of any new murmur found during routine clerking in patients aged 60 or over, particularly if the physical signs suggest *aortic stenosis*. Request an anesthetic review, following which surgery may well be delayed while echocardiography and/or a cardiology opinion is obtained.

5. Note any history of syncope, seizures, or repeated falls. Such patients may have a bradycardia, and any clinical diagnosis must be supported by an ECG as some uncommon conduction defects will need cardiological intervention before surgery.

6. Patients with undiagnosed or poorly controlled hypertension are a frequent cause of cancelled operations. Elucidate any other cardiac risk factors, measure the blood pressure in both arms, (recheck after the patient has had a period of rest; "white coat" hypertension is common), obtain an ECG, and await the decision of the anesthetist (a persistent diastolic pressure of 110 mm Hg or higher is generally accepted as needing preoperative treatment).

7. Patients taking warfarin require special consideration and are discussed in the section on *thromboprophylaxis*.

The Patient With a Pacemaker

In patients with a pacemaker, it is essential that prior to elective surgery you organize a 12-lead ECG, chest X-ray (CXR) and obtain the relevant old notes.

Unless done recently, the pacemaker function should be checked by cardiology technicians. Also, ensure that the responsible anesthetist and operating surgeon are aware and annotate the patient's theatre listing with the phrase "pacemaker in situ."

This advice is most pertinent with some of the modern pacemakers, which have a dual function as implantable defibrillators. *These devices must be inactivated before surgery and then reactivated as soon as possible thereafter*. This process requires the presence of a cardiology technician during the operative period.

Respiratory Disease

Patients with chronic obstructive pulmonary disease (COPD) are frequent in the population of individuals with a fractured neck of femur (NOF); younger patients with asthma are also not uncommon. The condition of patients with COPD can often be improved by attention to nebulizer therapy and treating any coexistent chest infection. A CXR is mandatory (particularly after a fall) to ensure that any other pulmonary pathology such as a pneumothorax or pleural effusion is not present. In addition to the routine investigations (delineated in this chapter), these patients' progress will often need to be monitored with arterial blood gases (take the sample while the patient breathes room air).

In all of the above, the input of the physiotherapist is crucial, and a respiratory physician's opinion may be necessary. The combined effort of the ward team can often significantly improve the physiological function of these patients before operation.

Asthmatic patients require care. Bronchospasm during general anesthesia is potentially lethal, and for all elective cases the patient's condition needs to be at a personal best. Always inquire specifically about asthma as it is remarkable how many stable asthmatic patients do not regard themselves as having a medical condition. Conversely, in severe cases, inquire specifically about current or recent steroid use. In patients describing recent deterioration have a low threshold for requesting a chest X-ray as "not all that wheezes is asthma."

Renal Disease
Patients with predialysis renal impairment are closely monitored by the renal physicians. The patients may have a restricted fluid intake, but prolonged preoperative starvation is also deleterious, and preoperatively intravenous fluids may be necessary.

Occasionally, dialysis-dependent renal inpatients are referred to the orthopedic team because of suspected joint sepsis or a fracture. These patients will be transferred to the orthopedic ward for surgery postdialysis. Following surgery, they will return to the renal unit for continuing dialysis. The opportunity for surgery occurs in a relatively small time frame. The most important issue here is communication. Ensure you are central in this and be certain regarding the whereabouts of the patient's notes and X-rays. Be prepared to discuss the case with the anesthetist and be certain of the patients postdialysis weight, hemoglobin, and potassium.

Neurology
Patients may present with neurological deficits because of injury or a variety of medical pathologies. Specific lesions (e.g., a radial nerve palsy) need careful documentation because any further postoperative neurological deterioration may be attributed to the surgery or anesthesia, with obvious medicolegal connotations.

Sickle Cell Status

Sickle cell status should be ascertained in any patient originating from Afro-Caribbean, African, and Mediterranean areas. The homozygous state is, of course, sickle cell disease; these patients would present with an established medical history. Of more practical importance is the heterozygous trait, which is not infrequent. Surgery can precipitate an ischemic crisis in these patients, particularly if tourniquets are involved.

Pregnancy

Patients of child-bearing age who are facing anesthesia or exposure to X-rays should be asked if there is any possibility of pregnancy. If there are any doubts, the women should be advised to have (with her consent) a pregnancy test. Obviously, there are situations in which these dictates must be applied with considerable sensitivity.

Occasionally, surgery will be necessary in a patient who is known to be pregnant. The anesthetist should be informed as early as possible. Depending on the stage of pregnancy, it may also be necessary to establish a liaison with obstetric colleagues so that perioperative fetal monitoring can be performed.

Drugs on Admission

For detailed information on prescribed medication, refer to the section Concurrent Medication.

Not all pharmacology is medically prescribed; concerns over alcohol or narcotic dependency should be referred for specialist assessment to minimize problems in the perioperative period.

In the preadmission clinic, female patients will often seek advice about the contraceptive pill and forthcoming surgery. Patients taking a low-dose progesterone-only pill can continue their contraception. The combined estrogen and progesterone preparations must either be stopped 4–6 weeks before surgery or heparin thromboprophylaxis given perioperatively. If the patient elects to discontinue the pill, she must be reminded of the need for alternative contraception; particularly, the risks of surgery in early pregnancy need to be emphasized.

Previous Anesthesia

1. Postoperative nausea and vomiting (PONV) is not uncommon and in a small percentage of patients causes significant short-term delay in recovery. Patients will often emphasize how they have previously suffered from what can be a debilitating problem. It is the anesthetist's responsibility to try to minimize any recurrence (although even when forewarned, this can be difficult).

2. *Suxamethonium apnea* is prolonged paralysis following a single dose of the otherwise short-acting muscle relaxant suxamethonium. The patient or a family member may have experienced this problem; annotate the patient's notes prior to the anesthetist's preoperative visit.
3. Rarely, the patient may offer a history of a relative who died or nearly died following general anesthesia for minor surgery. Many explanations are possible, including the very rare malignant hyperpyrexia. At the point of disclosure of such information, the priority is to personally inform the anesthetist who will be responsible for this patient; in the meanwhile, attempt to obtain any hospital notes relevant to the incident in question.

Latex Allergy

Allergy to the proteins found in natural rubber latex (NRL) has become a "fashionable" condition and includes patients who will claim that they are NRL sensitive despite repeated uneventful surgical episodes. The allergy may be documented after formal testing, but in the authors' experience it is usually the case that no such investigation has been performed.

Once declared, you need to inform the nursing staff and the surgeon responsible for constructing the operating list on which the patient will appear, then tell the theatre team. These patients will usually be placed first on the list as there are practical implications for both theatre and recovery. When writing the operating list, make sure the patient's sensitivity is documented.

With regard to your ward duties, you should:

1. Ensure all disposables (particularly gloves) are latex free. This may sound onerous, but most medical/nursing products are now manufactured latex free.
2. Take care with any latex-containing patient equipment (e.g., cover sphygmomanometer tubing).
3. Appropriately use latex-free dressings when siting intravenous infusions.
4. Administer drugs from glass ampoules or else ensure rubber bungs are removed.
5. If requesting investigations that involve exposure to other clinical areas (e.g., X-ray), inform the relevant department.

Routine Clinical Investigations

Routine clinical investigations are the baseline investigations used throughout medicine to measure or test basic clinical parameters (i.e., urinalysis, hemoglobin, urea, and electrolyte measurement; a 12- lead ECG; plain CXR).

In the United Kingdom, the National Institute for Clinical Excellence (NICE) has produced exhaustive recommendations for preoperative testing based on these four investigations and the patient's fitness and grade of surgery. In a similar strategy, the U.K. Royal College of Radiologists published guidelines on the requesting of preoperative CXRs (for both publications, see the Bibliography of this volume).

NICE graded surgery from 1 (minor) to 4 (major +); patient fitness is assessed using the American Society of Anesthesiologists (ASA) score. The ASA score is a functional assessment by which patients are classified as follows:

ASA 1: Normal healthy patient
ASA 2: Systemic medical condition (e.g., hypertension) that does not limit normal activity
ASA 3: Systemic medical condition that limits activity
ASA 4: Severe disease that is continually life threatening

Studying NICE's protocol, one is struck by the extensive use of the phrase "consider this test." This emphasizes the belief that investigations should be matched to the patient's health and the nature of the proposed surgery.

Despite the fact that fixed recommendations can never deal with every situation, your hospital may have "NICE-type" guidelines published as an in-house protocol; if so, follow it, *but* if in doubt about the wisdom of any investigation, ask.

In the history and examination section, we have indicated where we feel that an ECG or CXR is specifically required. More generally, you should recognize that:

1. ASA 1 patients under the age of 40 have no requirement for a CXR, ECG, or routine blood studies.
2. Patients receiving digoxin or thiazide diuretic therapy must have their electrolytes checked; significant hyponatremia and hypokalemia are unacceptable prior to surgery.
3. Patients who have had recent major surgery may be anemic. Further surgery may require a check of hemoglobin status.
4. Arterial blood gas analysis is frequently needed in patients with significant respiratory problems.

Elective Surgery and the Blood Transfusion Laboratory
Blood is a scarce resource, and transfusion is not without risks. The present trend is to minimize the need for blood products by a variety of strategies, including predonation, cell salvage techniques, and reduced transfusion triggers (i.e., accepting anemia).

Your hospital should have a local transfusion committee with its own **MSBOS** (maximum surgical blood order schedule) protocol that will match the surgical procedure and the number of units of concentrated red cells needed. Such protocols cannot fully anticipate variation in patients' physiological condition or surgical technique. As a consequence, when in doubt ask: Is a *group and save* (to identify the patient's ABO blood group/Rhesus type and test the sample for red cell antibodies) or an actual *cross match* (prepare units of compatible blood to be ready for that patient) required for this particular procedure?

Analysis of critical incidents during blood transfusion reveals the most common problem occurs because the "wrong unit of blood is given to the wrong patient." The root cause is misidentification of samples. When withdrawing blood, take the sample tube and request forms to the patient's bedside. It is imperative to ensure that sample tube and request form are completely and properly labeled (for the sample tube, always do this by hand and preferably likewise for the form). The patient's full name and date of birth must be confirmed by checking the patient's identity wristband.

Remember that a group-and-save request remains current for 5 days; any necessity for transfusion thereafter requires a fresh serum sample.

The aim of preoperative medical preparation is to identify actual or potential morbidity that needs correction and is correctable; subsequent clinical or laboratory investigations should reflect this.

FURTHER READING
In this chapter, see the section Concurrent Medication and Part II, Consent and Identification; also see Section 3, Special Patient Groups.

Concurrent Medication
An inevitable partner of the patient with chronic medical conditions is the patient's medication. Such medication can interact with anesthesia and surgery in both beneficial and negative manners.

Principles

1. A drug's therapeutic, protective, or prophylactic action may mean that its use should be continued throughout the perioperative period at the normal or possibly increased dosage.

2. A drug may have recognized negative interactions with anesthesia or surgery and should be discontinued or changed to another preparation before surgery.

Both Principles 1 and 2 may be influenced by the type and duration of surgery and whether it is elective or emergency.

3. When polypharmacy is an issue, the drugs must be prioritized before deciding what should be given on the morning of surgery.
4. A drug regarded as neutral in respect of Principles 1 and 2 can be safely omitted on the day of surgery as part of the "nothing by mouth" (NPO) status.
5. A patient's drug allergy or idiosyncratic reaction must be documented so those that might otherwise be given in the perioperative period can be avoided.

Practical Considerations
Your responsibility is to document the patient's medication on admission and record any declared allergies. In certain cases, ensuring accurate information will require contact with the patient's general practitioner. It is usual practice to initially prescribe the patient's normal regime and then make any subsequent adjustments or omissions according to perioperative needs.

An exception occurs if it is clearly necessary to make changes some time prior to planned surgery or immediately on hospital admission. In these instances, follow the instructions of your seniors or take advice from other specialists as necessary.

Drugs in the Perioperative Period
In Table 4.1, "can be omitted" refers to the wish to minimize preoperative oral intake in accordance with the policy of nothing by mouth. When it is considered necessary to take medication, the use of a small volume of water does not adversely affect this policy.

When patients are receiving special benefit from a small number of tablets or capsules, then unless there is an absolute contraindication, it is often better to give the medication with surgery.

FURTHER READING
All remaining parts of this chapter's Part I, Medical Preparation, should be consulted.

Fasting
As with any cause of decreased level of consciousness, anesthesia temporarily removes or reduces the protective reflexes around the

TABLE 4.1. Perioperative Drugs

Classification	Role in Anesthesia and Surgery
1. Corticosteroids	The physiological stress of intercurrent illness and surgery means that patients will require increased doses of *hydrocortisone* or *prednisolone* in the perioperative period. This may necessitate a period of intravenous dosing and subsequent staged reduction to the admission dose.
2. Anticoagulants	*Warfarin* must be discontinued before surgery and possibly substituted with heparin (see Thromboprophylaxis).
3. Antiplatelet agents	*Clopidogrel* and its relative *ticlopidine* are increasingly used by cardiologists and neurologists to prevent stent thrombosis and manage ischemia. The manufacturers recommend discontinuing the drug before elective surgery (fear of uncontrolled hemorrhage) (see Thromboprophylaxis).
	Aspirin may be stopped preoperatively or actively continued as thromboprophylaxis; there is no consensus regarding which approach is "correct."
	Dipyridamole need not be stopped.
4. Antihypertensives and treatment for heart failure	There is no absolute agreement, but most authorities believe that blood pressure control should be uninterrupted perioperatively.
	There is considerable evidence that *beta blockers* can protect against cardiac ischemia and sometimes are prescribed de novo before operation.
	The reduced plasma volume of the starved patient means that some anesthetists will want *diuretics* or *ACE (angiotensin-converting enzyme) inhibitors/angiotensin receptor antagonists* omitted on the day of surgery.
5. Angina treatment	Regular *nitrates* and *calcium channel blockers* should not be omitted. If the patient has a *GTN* spray, it should accompany them to the operating theater.
6. Antiarrhythmics	Treatment should *not* be withheld.

Continued

TABLE 4.1. Perioperative Drugs

Classification	Role in Anesthesia and Surgery
7. Statins	Statins should be maintained as there is increasing evidence that they have a cardio-protective effect.
8. Bronchodilators	Patients should be encouraged to use their own or prescribed *inhalers* as normal to minimize the potential hazard of bronchospasm during anesthesia. The same drugs may be prescribed in nebulized form as premedication. Inhalers should also accompany the patient to the operating theater.
9. Blood glucose control	*Oral hypoglycemics:* Omit on day of surgery (see The Diabetic Patient). *Insulin:* Regime will need to be adjusted according to nature and duration of surgery (see The Diabetic Patient)
10. Antireflux, antacids, proton pump inhibitors	Many anesthetists will want these drugs given on the day of surgery to minimize the risks of airway contamination. They may be prescribed as "premedication" or used postoperatively to minimize gastric side effects of aspirin and nonsteroidal anti-inflammatories (NSAIDs).
11. Antiepileptics	Should be maintained
12. Antimigraine	Should be given as soon as possible after surgery
13. Thyroxine	Should be maintained
14. Contraceptive pill	Patients may have had instructions to stop the drug preadmission; alternatively, thromboprophylaxis is prescribed (see discussion in Problems Identified During the History and Physical Examination).
15. Drugs used for Parkinson's disease	Can be omitted on day of surgery. Note: (a) If recently prescribed, they can contribute to postoperative confusion; (b) extrapyramidal complications may be seen with perioperative use of sedatives/antiemetics.
16. Immunosuppressants	Patients on these medications are likely to have a complicated medical history. A short interruption in treatment may be tolerated, but if in doubt get advice. Also see discussion of steroids in this table.

17. Analgesics	Most can be safely omitted on day of surgery as analgesia is "a given" with respect to subsequent surgery and postoperative period. However, be careful to ensure that patients with chronic pain receive all their normal dosage at least up to the morning of operation. A special situation is patients receiving *methadone* maintenance for a previous heroin addiction. Their normal daily dose must be regarded as a basic physiological requirement, and these patients should be referred to your drug dependency team. Some consultants will request that *NSAIDs* are not prescribed postoperatively as they can promote bleeding. They also have renal effects such that their use in elderly patients requires careful attention.
18. Antibiotics and antifungals	Antibiotics will often be given intravenously during surgery, while antifungals can be omitted before surgery (except for intravenous antifungals in the ill patient). These drugs are often long acting and can usually be safely omitted for short periods.
19. Antidepressants and antipsychotics	There is the potential for sedative and extrapyramidal interactions with postoperative analgesia and antiemetics. *Monoamine oxidase inhibitors* are used infrequently; they can produce cardiorespiratory depression with pethidine.
20. Hormone replacement therapy (HRT) and hormone antagonists	*HRT* or *raloxifene* may be discontinued before surgery (risk of venous thromboembolism) or maintained perioperatively under cover of thromboprophylaxis.

airway and lungs. Restricting food and fluid before anesthesia and surgery is an attempt to decrease gastric contents and so minimize the risk of them being aspirated into the lungs.

Fasting periods are based on historical studies of gastric emptying, and recently the accepted "nothing-by-mouth" period for elective patients has decreased. Each hospital usually has a fasting policy, but accepted general guidelines are as follows:

Food: 6 hours
Clear fluids: 2 hours

Clear fluids means that if the fluid was put in a glass, a newspaper could be read through the fluid. Clear fluids include water, apple juice, and tea without milk. They *DO NOT* include orange juice and cow's milk, which is regarded as a food.

"Sips" of water may be allowed closer to the operation, as are small quantities of water to take essential medications.

In principle, if the order of the operating list is known and the duration of the operations can be forecast by the surgeon, it is possible to tailor fasting times for individual patients. The reality is that due to the unpredictable and chaotic nature of operating theaters, the wards may operate a blanket nothing-by-mouth policy after a time, such as midnight or 2 a.m. The result is that some patients come to the operating theater unnecessarily hungry and thirsty. One laudable method of treatment is to establish a crystalloid infusion overnight (or during the day of surgery if events conspire to delay the patient's arrival in the operating theater); if so and if the surgery is an upper limb procedure, do site the cannula in the *nonoperative limb*.

Patients Who May Not Be Regarded as Starved."
1. Emergency patients who have suffered acute trauma. Here it is the interval between the last meal and time of injury that is important. Opiates given for pain relief will also slow gastric emptying.
2. Certain medical conditions (e.g., obesity, hiatal hernia, or diabetes) can (a) influence the mechanics of gastric emptying or (b) promote esophageal reflux, so these patients may also be considered as not being starved.
3. Beware chewing gum: Patients will not necessarily recognize this as "food," but studies showing that it increases gastric contents and pH have altered its status. Patient's day surgery preadmission letters often make this point explicit, but it still causes cancellations.

These are issues for the anesthetist and should not influence your routine preoperative preparation.

Modern studies indicated that in elective surgery clear fluids are safe up to 2 hours before operation.

FURTHER READING

In this chapter, see the section Concurrent Medication; also see Chapter 5, Intravenous Fluids and Electrolytes.

The Diabetic Patient

Diabetes mellitus results from a lack of insulin or from resistance to its action. In pathological terms, diabetes is a vascular disease, and this is reflected in many of its complications. Strict perioperative control of blood sugar reduces the risk of acute problems, including infection.

Traditionally, patients are classified as having the following types of diabetes:

1. Insulin-dependent diabetes mellitus (IDDM) = type 1. These patients will take regular subcutaneous injections of insulin, which will be prescribed in combinations of short- and medium-/long-acting preparations. The choice of insulin and the exact dosing regime will depend on the individual.
2. Non-insulin-dependent diabetes mellitus (NIDDM) = type 2. These patients are managed by a combination of diet or diet and oral hypoglycemics.

The sulfonylurea antidiabetic drugs are long acting and are often taken just once daily in the morning. The biguanide (metformin) may be taken either in isolation (three times a day) or with a sulfonylurea (e.g., glibenclamide). Newer antidiabetic drugs include the thiazolidnediones (which act by reducing peripheral insulin resistance); some patients will take these in combination with one of the other types (usually a sulfonylurea).

A small number of patients will take both insulin (generally as a bedtime dose) and oral hypoglycemics.

It is clear therefore that the traditional classification is an oversimplification; there is a continuum, from health to glycemic control with diet and medication, to total insulin dependence. This has implications for managing these patients perioperatively.

Diabetes and Surgery

Surgery and anesthesia cause a neuroendocrine stress response that raises blood glucose. The situation is worsened in any situation in which hypovolemia is significant. The greater the

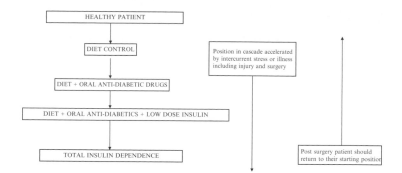

FIGURE 4.2. The surgical diabetic ladder.

physiological stress, the larger the disturbance in sugar homeostasis (Figure 4.2).

The management of the diabetic depends on their preexisting diabetic control and the type of surgery they face. The distinction between elective and emergency cases is also important.

Traditionally, diabetic patients are operated on early in the morning to minimize the starvation period. For day cases in particular, this allows early resumption of their normal regime and postoperative stabilization prior to discharge.

The most practical question to ask yourself is: Is it expected that this patient will be eating and drinking normally after the surgery? This translates to missing only one meal (breakfast). The answer to this question should be yes for *all* day cases and a large number of inpatient procedures.

The aim is to disturb their normal regime as little as possible; protocols for elective surgery (which respects the "only-one-missed-meal rule") are outlined in Table 4.2.

Sliding Scale Insulin
The principle of sliding scale insulin is that the patient is managed throughout the perioperative period by an intravenous infusion of 5% dextrose and short-acting insulin until such time as their general medical condition permits them to return to their normal subcutaneous insulin requirements. The infusions are started preoperatively and monitored by regular blood glucose measurements, aiming to maintain a blood glucose of 6–9 mmol/L.

All hospitals should have protocols for initiating and managing sliding scale regimes, including guidance on what actions to take in the event of hypoglycemia or persistent hyperglycemia.

TABLE 4.2. Diabetic Patient Perioperative Protocol

	Day Case or Minor/ Intermediate Inpatient	Major: Inpatient
IDDM, type 1	Omit their breakfast insulin preoperatively and postoperatively supply a proportion of their morning insulin dose with their first postoperative meal. Thereafter, their normal regime continues, and any small increase in insulin dose will often be patient managed. Their normal evening insulin is given the night before surgery, and early the following morning the intravenous regime is commenced.	Even though they may be able to eat and drink postoperatively, these patients are often best managed in the first instance using a sliding scale regime (see next section) of intravenous insulin.
NIDDM, type 2	On the day of surgery, any oral hypoglycemics are omitted presurgery and the usual dose given with their first postoperative food.	In principle, intravenous insulin should be avoidable, but a proportion of cases will require it. Others may require temporary subcutaneous insulin.

Emergency Surgery

Patients for emergency surgery will often have elevated blood sugar on admission, and in some instances their diabetes will be directly contributing to the need for surgical admission. To achieve satisfactory glycemic control, sliding scale insulin will often be required.

Complications and Difficult Cases

Various problems can frustrate diabetic control. Beware of the following:

1. Postoperative vomiting from whatever cause may prevent the otherwise straightforward day case patient from being managed as described. In such cases, as soon as it is clear that normal oral intake is going to be significantly delayed, then the patient will need switching to a sliding scale regime.

2. In an attempt to minimize PONV, anesthetists may manage diabetic patients with regional anesthesia. Their enthusiasm for this can be influenced by the presence of diabetic neuropathy, and your preoperative clerking should attempt to identify any known neurological deficit.

3. Patients with poorly controlled diabetes scheduled for elective surgery should be deferred until their condition is stabilized. Should you identify such a patient who has been admitted for operation, inform the responsible anesthetist at the first opportunity.

4. Intravenous insulin decreases serum potassium, which may need monitoring. Your sliding scale protocol should contain instructions for potassium supplementation. Be particularly aware of those patients also receiving diuretics.

5. The infusion rates prescribed by your sliding scale protocol may need to be increased by up to two to four times in sick patients; this includes steroid-dependent individuals. If the blood glucose is persistently elevated (>15 mmol/L), the 5% dextrose will need to be substituted with normal saline and expert help sought.

6. Following major surgery and resumption of normal oral intake and the usual daily subcutaneous insulin dose, some patients will have a transition period in which blood glucose remains elevated. These cases are managed by a temporary increase in their insulin dosage. This may require changing the frequency and type of insulin given; such cases should be referred to and managed under the instructions of a diabetologist.

7. Similarly, patients with type 2 diabetes who require temporary subcutaneous insulin will also benefit from specialist input.

> Strict perioperative control of blood glucose in type 1 diabetics needing major surgery will inevitably require intravenous insulin.

FURTHER READING
See all other sections of Part I, Medical Preparation, and Chapter 5, Intravenous Fluids and Electrolytes.

Thromboprophylaxis
Orthopedic patients are at particular risk of thromboembolic complications. Relevant factors include prolonged operative procedures and immobility secondary to traction, plaster casts, or splints. Associated factors include the following:

1. Obesity and smoking
2. The contraceptive pill in combination with surgery
3. Preexisting malignant disease
4. Dehydration
5. Elderly patients
6. Patients with a previous history of thromboembolism

Patient History
Particular note should be made of any of the precipitating or complicating factors listed. You should inquire about any previous history of deep venous thrombosis (DVT) or pulmonary embolism (PE); a positive response must be clearly recorded in the patient's notes.

During any inpatient admission, thromboprophylactic drugs are likely to be prescribed; it is therefore imperative that note is taken of any *current medication for which bleeding is acknowledged to be a complication (e.g., warfarin, clopidogrel, aspirin).*

Techniques for Thromboprophylaxis
The aim of thrombophrophylaxis is to minimize stasis in the deep veins and hence prevent development of clots. Immobilization for as little as 1–2 days is sufficient for the onset of thromboembolic complications.

Techniques may be used in isolation or combination and include the following:
Ensuring adequate hydration, including preoperative intravenous
  infusion
Use of elastic stockings
Use of calf compression devices intra- and postoperatively
Early postoperative mobilization and physiotherapy
Pharmacology: Use of thromboprophylactic medication usually
  starts preoperatively and is routinely maintained throughout
  the perioperative period

Drugs Used for Thromboprophylaxis
A large number of drugs affect either the coagulation cascade or platelet function. They include:

1. Warfarin.
2. Unfractionated (or standard) heparin; this is quick acting but of short duration. It is given intravenously as a loading dose followed by an infusion. The effect on coagulation must be monitored by daily measurement of the activated partial thromboplastin time (APPT).
3. Low molecular weight heparin (LMWH) is longer acting compared to standard heparin and is given once daily by

subcutaneous injection; laboratory monitoring is not required. Examples are enoxaparin (20–40 mg daily) and dalteparin (2,500 units daily).
4. Platelet inhibitors such as aspirin, NSAIDs, dipyridamole, and clopidogrel.
5. Newer drugs such as fondaparinux, which is a synthetic pentasaccharide recently licensed for prophylaxis in major orthopedic surgery.

There is no universal agreement among orthopedic surgeons regarding which of these drugs are best used for operative thromboprophylaxis or indeed which of them need to be withdrawn before surgery to minimise hemorrhage.

The Patient on Long-Term Warfarin

Patients with valvular heart disease or atrial fibrillation or who have suffered a recent (within the last 6 months) thromboembolic event will already be taking warfarin. Warfarin is normally given as a loading dose of 10 mg daily for 2 days, followed by a daily maintenance dose of 3–9 mg, which is adjusted by monitoring the international normalized ratio (INR). The patient's target INR will reflect his or her underlying condition and will range between 2.0 and 3.5.

Warfarin is long acting and also interacts with many drugs; hence, the usual practice during the perioperative period is to change the warfarin to shorter-acting alternatives. The exact way in which this is done will vary according to the patient's medical condition and the nature of the proposed surgery.

Recognized regimes include:
Elective surgery

1. Stop warfarin 3 days before surgery (ideally, this should be done in consultation with the patient's general practitioner and the anticoagulant clinic).
2. Check INR on the morning of surgery; it should be in the range 1.5–2.0.
3. The perioperative period may be covered by LMWH, an intravenous heparin infusion, or neither depending on the situation for that individual patient. Any heparin infusion must be commenced, stopped, and restarted at safe intervals dictated by two estimates: (a) the start time of surgery (stop infusion 4 hours before) and (b) the end of the early postoperative period, during which hemorrhage is a real risk (around 12 hours).
4. When the risk of immediate postoperative hemorrhage has passed, the patient is reloaded with warfarin and subsequently returned to their usual maintenance dose. This process, which

is monitored by checking the INR, will take between 48 and 72 hours. During this period, high-risk patients will continue their alternative anticoagulation.

Emergency Surgery: The defined aim is for surgery within 12–24 hours, and in the orthopedic context this is especially relevant to the fractured NOF patients, for whom operative delay is clearly associated with increased mortality. In this situation:

1. Stop warfarin and reverse action with intravenous vitamin K (1 mg).
2. Check INR before operating as discussed; desirable range is 1.5–2.0.
3. If INR unacceptable at 24 hours (it is a common observation that after stopping the warfarin the INR rises before eventually falling), a further dose of vitamin K can be given.
4. Consideration can be given to providing additional cover with fresh frozen plasma (initial dose = 10–15 mL/kg).
5. When the INR is less than 2.0, consider the need for alternative thromboprophylaxis.
6. Postoperative management is the same as for the elective status.

Clopidogrel

Clopidogrel works by inhibiting platelet aggregation and is in increasing use by physicians to manage ischemic vascular conditions, including thromboprophylaxis in coronary stents. Once discontinued, its antiplatelet effects continue for 24 hours. Current U.K. experience suggests that a reasonable perioperative approach is as follows:

Elective surgery: Discontinue 7 days before surgery.

Emergency surgery: If possible, discontinue for 24 hours and then proceed (platelet transfusion may be required). This advice is once again seen as being particularly relevant to NOF patients.

The complicating factor is those patients with coronary stents; here, the overall risks of stopping clopidogrel will depend on the type of stent (drug-eluting stents require longer treatment with clopidogrel) and the insertion particulars—surgery interval and stent location (proximal versus distal). Prior to surgery, discuss particulars of these patients with the relevant cardiologist.

The risk of postoperative hemorrhage is clearly increased in the presence of anticoagulation (particularly with a heparin infusion), and this combined with an individual patient's history plus the nature of the surgery mitigate against a "standard thromboprophylactic prescription."

In practice, successful management of difficult cases, such as a patient who has suffered from recurrent DVT, will require consultation with a hematologist.

Dosing of Anticoagulant Drugs and Spinal/Epidural Anesthesia

Spinal and epidural anesthesia are themselves associated with a decreased risk of thromboembolic complications (as compared to general anesthesia), but that is not the issue here. You need to be aware that a complication of either technique (but particularly epidurals) includes epidural hematoma, epidural abscess, and meningitis.

The possibility of causing an epidural hematoma is increased in the presence of anticoagulation, so that the time interval between giving the anticoagulant and performing the epidural is important. The same is true for subsequent removal of an epidural catheter.

The "safe" time to perform either procedure relies on there being a point at which the anticoagulant effect of the drug will be minimal, and this in turn is dependant on its pharmacology.

Reasonable guidelines (definitive evidence-based guidelines do not exist) are given in Table 4.3 for information. It is the responsibility of the anesthetist to ensure that these criteria are met if he or she is contemplating a central neural block.

Table 4.3 implies that central neural blockade can be successfully associated with subsequent heparin infusion. This requires rigorous attention to detail, and should you come across such a situation, you should expect the responsible anesthetist to be closely involved in postoperative management. Another occasion when you might expect anesthetic supervision postoperatively is if the epidural was technically difficult and might have been associated with bleeding.

TABLE 4.3. Dosing Guidelines for Anticoagulant Drugs and Spinal/Epidural Anesthesia

Drug	Procedure: Dose interval
Aspirin	No special consideration required
Unfractionated heparin, subcutaneous	Give heparin either 4 hours preprocedure or 2 hours postprocedure
LMWH, subcutaneous	Give heparin 12 hours before siting epidural or 2 hours after catheter removal
Unfractionated heparin infusion, intravenous	Commence 12 hours postepidural insertion. Do not remove epidural catheter until 4 hours after stopping infusion and only after checking that APPT and platelet count are normal.
Warfarin	INR must be less than 1.5 before procedure.

Symptoms and Signs of Spinal Cord Compression

The classical signs suggestive of a spinal cord problem result from the subsequent cord compression.

Epidural abscesses and meningitis occur around 5 days after removal of the epidural catheter, while epidural hematomas tend to develop while the catheter is still in situ.

Early clues include difficulty in micturition, localized back pain, and leg weakness. Leg weakness is assessed by starting at the toes and assessing in turn ankle, knee, and finally hip flexion. Scored and compare both legs for weakness.

Spinal cord compression is an emergency; see the section in this chapter Managing Suspected Cord Compression.

The Patient With Neurology and an Epidural In Situ

For the patient with neurology and an epidural in situ, this means either increasing anesthesia (or symptoms discussed in the preceding section), which is *not* obviously accounted for by a recent active change in the epidural such as an increase in the prescribed dose or a change to a higher concentration of local anesthetic.

Any progressive sensorimotor deficit or sphincter disturbance is an important sign suggesting the onset of a spinal hematoma, which is easily missed or attributed to the "success" of the epidural. Likewise, in this situation back pain must not be discounted as musculoskeletal.

This may mean spinal cord compression; see the next section in this chapter, Managing Suspected Cord Compression.

Managing Suspected Cord Compression

At the first suggestion of inappropriate neurology, *stop* the epidural infusion if still running and call the pain team immediately; *make it clear why you are seeking their assistance. Do not remove the epidural catheter.* At the same time, *inform* your own seniors and do not let the patient receive anything by mouth. If an epidural hematoma is suspected, an emergency magnetic resonance imaging (MRI) scan will be indicated; if the diagnosis is confirmed, emergency decompression will follow.

Speed is essential as decompression needs to be performed within *8 hours* of the onset of symptoms. By the time a sensorimotor level is established with paralysis below this level, the situation is usually permanent.

Safe perioperative thromboprophylaxis depends on understanding the pharmacology of the anticoagulants involved.

FURTHER READING
See the section Concurrent Medication in this chapter and Chapter 13, Deep Venous Thrombosis and Pulmonary Embolism.

PART II: CONSENT AND IDENTIFICATION
A core function of a surgical unit is to get patients safely through their operation and home again. While the medical preparation described is central to initiating this process, the next critical steps are to ensure that:
1. The patient understands what is being proposed and why
2. Subsequently, that the correct operation is performed on the right patient

Consent for Elective Surgery
Consent for elective surgery is always best undertaken either by the operating surgeon or an experienced registrar. On occasions, it will be your responsibility. The following statements are reasonable guidelines:

1. Do not offer information on technique, risks, or complications that you cannot substantiate from either personal experience or evidence base.
2. Always give the patient an opportunity to ask questions; do not rush consent taking.
3. Answer questions truthfully, and if you do not know an answer, say so.
4. If the patient requests information outside of your knowledge or experience, refer upward; never pressure them into signing.
5. Always pitch your descriptions and explanations such that they are comprehensible to the patient.
6. Keep your descriptions of the risks of the procedure within practical limits; for instance, mentioning thromboembolic complications during consent for knee replacement is clearly mandatory, while discussing septicemia from insertion of the preoperative intravenous cannula (theoretically reasonable) is not helpful.
7. A good way to conclude is simply to ask: Is there any part of our discussion that you wish to challenge or have explained further?

Consent in Difficult Situations
Certain situations are potential medical-legal minefields. The following examples are not uncommon:

1. *Emergency surgery:* Here, the same principles outlined apply, but time may be an issue.
2. *The incompetent patient:* This may occur because of physical or mental health problems. Sometimes, the difficulty here can be dealing with relatives or caregivers.
3. *Specific patient groups* such as Jehovah Witnesses, who will refuse specific treatments.

When such situations present, your role in obtaining consent will become one of a coordinator. As soon as it is clear that the situation is not straightforward, inform your seniors and await guidance. Purpose-designed consent forms are available for certain situations, but on rare occasions specific legal guidance may have to be obtained. This is time consuming and reinforces the need for early referral.

A complete treatment of the ethical considerations required in obtaining consent are available online from the U.K. General Medical Council (see the Bibliography this volume).

Anesthesia: Consent and Practical Issues
Undergraduate knowledge of anesthesia is not assumed when you take on the foundation year role; also, separate written consent is not routinely obtained for anesthesia. The following notes will hopefully assist:

1. If the patient declares a previous anesthetic mishap, make it clear that avoiding a repetition on this occasion is the responsibility of the anesthetist, who will visit the patient before surgery. Thereafter, proceed as outlined in the notes on previous anesthesia (in this chapter, see the history and physical examination information in Part I, Medical Preparation).
2. Never assume that an "unfit" patient (with significant medical comorbidity) will have surgery performed under a regional or local anesthetic technique. In particular, never assume that hip or lower limb surgery in such patients requires spinal anesthesia.
3. As a consequence of Note 2, never take it on yourself to tell the patient what type of anesthesia the patient will receive. If a patient asks you directly, point out that this will be discussed at the anesthetist's preoperative visit. The exception to this rule applies if you work in a unit (e.g., hand surgery) where standard protocols apply, such that normally all the patients receive exactly the same anesthetic (such as a specific regional technique). Even in this situation, do not volunteer information

to the patient until you are completely familiar with the unit's methods.

4. If it has been decided that a patient is to receive a local or regional anesthetic, ensure that they are still medically prepared as for general anesthesia.

5. Until told otherwise, keep all surgical patients (irrespective of type of anesthesia) restricted to nothing by mouth for the appropriate period.

6. Premedication: Do not premedicate patients unless under instruction.

7. If the anesthetists decide that a postoperative high-dependency unit (HDU) or intensive care unit (ICU) bed is required, double check that this has indeed been booked, and that the other members of your team are aware of the intended postoperative location. Visit the unit in question and find out what, if any, input is required from you when the patient is admitted.

8. Finally, if unsure or in need of advice find the responsible anesthetist and ask.

Identification for Surgery: Correct Patient for the Correct Operation

Increasingly, identification of the correct patient for the correct operation is handled by the operating surgeon, but the safe principles should be understood by all doctors. This is part of the necessary preoperative checklists performed by the ward and theater staff.

The process requires that:

1. Printed operating lists identify both the surgeon responsible for care and the surgeon operating on that patient.

2. Every patient on the operating list should be *named fully* and identified with a *unit number* and *date of birth*.

3. Should two patients on the same list have the same name, this must be made very clear, for example, with the words "Warning: Two patients on the list with same surname" written conspicuously.

4. Operative descriptions should be comprehensive, unambiguous, and devoid of abbreviations.

5. Operating on the incorrect side (wrong-site surgery) is rare, but there is evidence from medical indemnity claims that its prevalence is actually rising: *Right* and *Left* must be written as such, *not* R or L.

6. The limb must be marked. In bilateral procedures, the marks should be annotated. For example, make it clear that the right knee is for cruciate ligament reconstruction, while the left is only a diagnostic arthroscopy.

7. The procedure the patient has *consented to* and that on the *operating list* must match.
8. You do not change a submitted list once operating has begun without first informing the operating surgeon, anesthetist, and appropriate theater team.

In aviation and in high-performance industrial processes, one of the core tenets is that anyone can draw attention to a potential problem that may lead to an error without fear of recrimination. This culture needs to increasingly translate to surgical team practice.

Although rare the incidence of wrong site surgery is increasing.

FURTHER READING

See Part I, Medical Preparation, in this chapter.

Chapter 5
Intravenous Fluids and Electrolytes

Many orthopedic patients will only require intravenous fluids for a short time, if at all. Unlike a general surgical ward, oral intake is normally only restricted for short periods. In practice, you will find intravenous fluids are needed:

1. Prophylactically, to minimize dehydration in fasting patients awaiting surgery.
2. To maintain normal fluid balance in the small number of patients for whom the normal oral route is temporarily lost or requires supplementation (e.g., some vulnerable or confused patients with a fractured neck of femur). Some of these patients will be significantly dehydrated on admission following a lengthy recumbency before discovery by friends or relatives.
3. For blood transfusion pre- or postsurgery.
4. For volume restoration as part of resuscitation. Although common in the emergency department and the operating theater, this should be a rare event on the ward.

FLUIDS USED IN ROUTINE PRACTICE
Rational choice of fluids requires an understanding of physiology, injury processes, and fluid characteristics. The adult patient has a daily requirement for the following:

- Water: 40 mL/kg
- Na^+: 1–2 mmol/kg
- K^+: 0.5–1 mmol/kg

A fluid that is isotonic with plasma exerts the same osmotic pressure because the concentration of its solutes is equivalent.

- A *crystalloid* solution is an aqueous solution of electrolytes or other water-soluble molecules.
- A *colloid* is a suspension of large molecules in a carrier solution.

P. Wood et al., *Trauma and Orthopedic Surgery in Clinical Practice*,
DOI: 10.1007/978-1-84800-339-2_5, © Springer-Verlag London Limited 2009

Broadly speaking, intravenous fluids can be classified as:

1. Isotonic crystalloids (same tonicity as body fluids)
2. Artificial colloids used for volume expansion
3. Hypertonic crystalloids (greater tonicity than body fluids)
4. Blood (a natural colloid) and blood products (i.e., blood and derived components)

Isotonic Crystalloids

The main isotonic crystalloid fluids used to replace maintenance losses are 0.9% saline and lactated Ringer's (Hartmann's) solution. They are distributed throughout the extracellular fluid (so if used for resuscitation, approximately three times the volume of crystalloid is required to replace an equivalent volume of blood loss).

The 5% dextrose is iso-osmolar with plasma, but the dextrose is rapidly metabolized, creating free water, which is distributed throughout the body. Stronger solutions of dextrose (e.g., 10%, 20%, and 50%) are used to correct hypoglycemia.

The contents of a 1-L bag of the commonly used crystalloids are given in Table 5.1 (also see Figure 5.1).

Artificial Colloids

Artificial colloids include dextrans (chains of glucose units), starches, and gelatins. The large colloid molecules are suspended in crystalloid solution, and intravenous infusion increases the osmotic pressure within the blood vessels. Their duration of action varies with the size of the molecules and how the body processes them.

Colloid preparations are more expensive than crystalloids and can be associated with complications such as allergic reactions and interference with cross matching and coagulation.

TABLE 5.1. Commonly Used Crystalloid Compositions

	0.9% Saline (Normal Saline)	Hartmann's Solution (Lactated Ringers)	0.18% Saline + 4% Dextrose (Dextrose Saline)	5% Dextrose
Water (liters)	1	1	1	1
Na$^+$ (mmol)	150	130	30	
Cl$^-$ (mmol)	150	109	30	
K$^+$ (mmol)		4		
Ca^{2+} (mmol)		1.5		
Lactate (mmol)		28		
Glucose (g)			40	50

Product code number   Volume (ml)

Manufacturers name

Fluid identification

e.g. **Sodium Chloride Intravenous Infusion 0.9% W/V**

Viaflex ® container

-Sterile nonpyrogenic   solution for infusion
-Single dose

Each 1000 mi contains   **mmol/1000 ml (approx)**

Solute contents (in grms)   electrolyte concentrations
+ water for injections
+ osmolarity and pH

For intravenous administration
= instructions for storage.
pre infusion checks, and
iv admin

Manufacturers   Batch data   **POM**
address   = prescription only
                                          medicine
Lot no   Expiry date

Volume
indicator

FIGURE 5.1. What are you prescribing? Information displayed on the front of a bag of intravenous crystalloid (exact format will vary with manufacturer).

Hypertonic Crystalloids

When hypertonic saline is given intravenously, it draws fluid from the spaces between cells. The result is a rapid expansion of the intravascular volume for a short time.

Hypertonic saline Dextran (HSD) is a combination of 7.5% saline and Dextran 70, a colloid. The intention of this combination is that while hypertonic saline draws fluid into the blood vessels, the Dextran keeps this fluid within the vessels for a longer period than if hypertonic saline were used on its own.

Although these products apparently have certain key advantages (particularly in respect to resuscitation), they are not used routinely.

Blood and Blood Products

The blood transfusion service accepts a unit of donated blood and then separates it into its components. This maximizes use of the blood, and patients benefit from receiving exactly what their medical problem dictates.

The separation process produces red cells, plasma (containing clotting factors), albumin solutions, and individual clotting preparations such as factor 8.

"Packed cells" are red blood cells separated from the plasma after blood donation. These 300-mL (approximate volume) bags are what normally constitutes a "unit" of blood and are used to increase hemoglobin (i.e., oxygen-carrying capacity).

FLUID MANAGEMENT: SOME PRACTICAL OBSERVATIONS

1 If a patient can eat and drink, then let them.
2. The normal adult daily fluid requirement is 40 mL/kg; respect differences in body weight.
3. The *volume* of maintenance fluid you prescribe must equal:

Normal Daily Requirement + Extra insenible Losses + Electrolyte Requirements

These calculations are usually straightforward on the orthopedic ward as gastrointestinal function is not affected, but the "general surgical" approach to iintravenous fluids may be needed in:

   a. Patients with pelvic fractures and associated retroperitoneal hematoma
   b. Occasional instances of prolonged nausea and vomiting.

4. Your *choice* of intravenous fluid must answer the question, What effect is needed from the fluid?" (e.g., volume expansion vs. maintenance).
5. Respect the *rate* of fluid replacement; careful correction of perioperative dehydration is not the same exercise as rapid volume restoration in resuscitation. In particular, do not attempt rapid correction of sodium levels (see Table 5.2).
6. The effects of the metabolic response to trauma or surgery and any subsequent fluid administration must be monitored as with any other prescription. This requires clinical and charted assessment of intake versus output supplemented with serial checking and recording of hemoglobin, electrolytes, urea, and creatinine.

TABLE 5.2. Sodium and Potassium Disturbances

Electrolyte	Problem	Causes	Symptoms, Signs, Comments, Treatment
Sodium 135–150 mm/L	Hyponatremia	1. Dilutional from water intoxication (i.e., 5% dextrose infusion) 2. Thiazide + loop diuretics 3. Vomiting or diarrhea 4. Steroid deficiency 5. Exaggerated antidiuretic hormone (ADH) stress response	Malaise, headache, nausea and vomiting, confusion, convulsions, and coma possible at dangerous levels (<125 mm/L). Inappropriate 5% overload must be treated with strict fluid restriction. Most cases in an orthopedic ward will occur in euvolemic patients; the exception is severe diarrhea and vomiting. Note that principal action of ADH is to retain body water; therefore, inappropriate increased ADH perpetuates the problem. One rare cause of inappropriate increased ADH secretion is associated with pneumonia.
	Hypernatremia	1. Hypertonic saline infusion 2. Increased insensible losses	Note that elderly patients have a decreased "thirst response." 5% dextrose *may* be indicated, but usually for short periods only.
Potassium 3.5–5.2 mm/L	Hypokalemia	1. Thiazide + loop diuretics 2. Diarrhea or vomiting 3. Diabetic ketoacidosis 4. Insulin infusion 5. β-Adrenergic agonists - salbutamol 6. Alcoholics	Severe hypokalemia is associated with muscle weakness and occasionally cardiac arrhythmias. Electrocardiogram (ECG) may show prolonged QT interval, ST depression, flattened T waves and U waves. If K^+ > 3 mmol/L but needs supplementing, use oral effervescent preps (2–4 g daily)

(Continued)

TABLE 5.2. (Continued)

Electrolyte	Problem	Causes	Symptoms, Signs, Comments, Treatment
	Hyperkalemia	1. Renal insufficiency 2. Digitalis toxicity 3. Inappropriate K^+ prescriptions 4. Hemolysis during venipuncture or transport sample	If K^+ < 3 mm/L, intravenously supplement with a replacement rate not greater than 20–40 mmol/hour. Principal danger is cardiac—as K^+ increases, T wave peaking is followed by broad P waves and widening ST complexes—uncorrected, dangerous ventricular arrhythmias will supervene. Correction of renal causes must be directed at root cause. If K^+ is unexpectedly high, suspect sample haemolysis and carefully repeat. If K^+ is confirmed as greater than 7 mmol/L, give immediate intravenous calcium gluconate (10 mL 10%). Start infusion of 50 mL 50% dextrose plus 10 units actrapid insulin (over 15 min) while awaiting urgent medical opinion.

Notes: The postoperative patient is subject to a number of stress responses and attempts at homeostatic maintenance; the end result is that fluid and electrolyte disturbances can arise for which there is no obvious cause. Help may be required from a clinical biochemist, particularly in cases of hyponatremia. The response to either careful observation or active treatment must be monitored with serial measurements until the problem is resolved.

8. *Do not* routinely prescribe 5% dextrose as a recurring maintenance fluid because water intoxication, significant hyponatremia, confusion, and convulsions can easily arise. Similar unmonitored use of normal saline may result in elevated sodium.
9. Pay careful attention to patients taking diuretics. These drugs cause sodium and potassium loss in the urine, which is easily exacerbated by using the wrong fluids for maintenance therapy.
10. In elderly patients, beware of the dangers of acute volume overload and adjust maintenance requirements by body weight. This comment is not, however, an invitation for the routine use of diuretics when transfusing elderly patients. This practice is unnecessary.
11. If a patient has known renal disease requiring medical supervision of fluid intake, then fluids may need to be prescribed with the renal physician's advice.

SODIUM AND POTASSIUM DISTURBANCES ON THE ORTHOPEDIC WARD

Table 5.2 provides information on sodium and potassium disturbances on the orthopedic ward.

Fluid administration must respect normal physiology and the patient's current needs.

FURTHER READING

See the following: Chapter 4, the section Fasting; Chapter 8, The Patient With a Fractured Neck of Femur; Chapter 16, The Ill Patient and Medical Emergencies; and Chapter 17, Problems With Blood Transfusion.

Chapter 6
Analgesia

You will deal with analgesia in relation to three types of patient:

1. Patients admitted to the ward with acute injuries
2. Patients admitted to the ward for elective surgery who use regular analgesia because of chronic degenerative conditions, such as osteoarthritis or because of persistent pain following injury
3. Postoperative patients

Patients with acute injury will require timely control of their symptoms using suitable methods as listed here. Patients taking analgesics "long term" will often be under the care of the chronic pain clinic, and their medication is regarded as a physiological requirement. On admission, it is necessary to continue their usual regime before elective surgery, and postoperatively such patients will often be managed by specialized techniques discussed in this chapter.

Pain control in postoperative patients is overall a mixed bag; the patient's history, current analgesia, the type and duration of surgery, and anesthetic technique are all contributing factors, and at some point most of the discussion in this chapter will be relevant.

You will both prescribe and act as a monitor for other people's prescriptions, including techniques that are not necessarily taught to undergraduates. You will be assisted and guided in this process by the acute pain team.

What follows is a practical guide to help you in this aspect of your work.

ASSESSMENT OF PAIN
Descriptive scales are used to try to quantify a person's pain and gauge their response to treating it. In adults, you will find the use of a numeric intensity scale (e.g., 0–10 with 0 = no pain, 10 = worst pain imaginable) commonly used. Such scales do have limitations,

P. Wood et al., *Trauma and Orthopedic Surgery in Clinical Practice*,
DOI: 10.1007/978-1-84800-339-2_6, © Springer-Verlag London Limited 2009

but it is the overall trend following treatment that is important. Objective assessment aside, remember that pain is "what the patient says it is."

METHODS OF TREATING PAIN

Be aware that modern opinion is clear regarding the advantages of multimodal therapy. This means treating pain by a number of differing methods in combination as opposed to relying on one single drug or technique. It relies on acknowledging the fact that pain is consciously perceived only after a noxious stimulus has been received at the site of injury and then channeled and modulated at different areas and levels within the central nervous system. Successful pain control is achieved by disrupting this process at multiple locations. Treatment can be summarized as the 3 P's:

1. Psychological: Reassurance and concern for the patient's welfare
2. Physical: Splintage, traction, elevation, ice packs
3. Pharmacological: Simple analgesics, opiates, and local anesthetics

Analgesic drugs can be given by a variety of routes, but oral, intramuscular, rectal, and sublingual administration are standard. The intravenous route is used in three ways:

1. By bolus injection of morphine or a synthetic opiate. This is given in small divided doses until initial control of acute pain has been achieved. A common strategy in the emergency department or the postoperative recovery area, it may also be needed on the ward to "rescue" failed analgesia.
2. By patient-controlled analgesia (PCA). The apparatus for PCA allows maintenance of the benefit achieved by bolus injection. The patient injects him- or herself directly into a vein from a reservoir of opiate (usually morphine). The PCA apparatus is designed and set up so that the patient can only give a standard dose within a prescribed time frame (e.g., 1 mg of morphine every 5 min), thus preventing inappropriate usage. The cassettes used in these machines record their dispensations and incorporate various alarms. Their functioning should be routinely checked as a daily task of the acute pain team.
3. Fixed dosing of drugs that are more often given orally (e.g., paracetamol).

Simple Analgesics

Pharmacological treatment is escalated as necessary in a stepwise analgesic ladder, of which paracetamol and nonsteroidal anti-inflammatories (NSAIDs) (e.g., diclofenac and ibuprofen) tend to be the bottom tier. They are often prescribed in combination and are particularly effective in musculoskeletal injury. It is commonly stated that NSAIDs can worsen asthma. In our experience, this is very rare, but it is undeniable that they can interfere with hemorrhage and depress renal function. They must be avoided in cases of active gastric or duodenal ulcer or hypotensive patients. Even relatively short-term perioperative use can cause gastric irritation, particularly in elderly patients. Some orthopedic surgeons feel that they also negatively influence postoperative wound healing and will wish to avoid them for this reason.

Opiates

Traditionally, intramuscular opiate injection was the mainstay of postoperative analgesia. This approach, which often fails because of variable absorption and insufficient frequency of dosing, has been superseded by newer methods, including the oral use of morphine or synthetic opiates and intravenous PCA. Morphine is the standard PCA opiate, but pethidine is an alternative.

The biggest failure with opiates is their association with nausea and vomiting. This can severely limit their usefulness in some patients and encourages the use of other drugs to limit the total dose of morphine, hence the phrase "morphine sparing." Respiratory depression, confusion, sedation, constipation, itching, and urinary retention are other problems that can be particularly troublesome in the elderly. Constipation is also seen with prolonged usage of oral codeine (which works by hepatic conversion to morphine), which is often prescribed in combination with paracetamol and an NSAID.

Local Anesthetics

Local anesthetics are given for analgesia as infiltration, nerve blocks, and continuous catheter techniques. When used as local infiltration, they help to reduce the amount of systemic analgesics, and a few orthopedic procedures can be done entirely by this method.

Individual nerve or plexus blocks are undertaken to provide analgesia/anesthesia with or without associated general anesthesia. On occasions, indwelling catheters can be inserted around particular nerves to maintain anesthesia postoperatively using infusion pumps or by substituting local anesthetic for morphine in a PCA.

The most common type of indwelling catheter, however, is epidural. In these patients, postoperative analgesia is maintained with a continuous local anesthetic infusion that may also contain an opiate.

Any such infusions will also be reviewed and troubleshooting will be provided by the acute pain team.

PROBLEMS ASSOCIATED WITH ANALGESIA

Understandably, problems associated with analgesia result as a direct effect of the pharmacology of the drug involved. Unwanted effects can (and frequently are) worsened by the patient's overall physiological status. Although some complications can be life threatening (e.g., respiratory depression), it is often the less-serious effects that patients find intolerable. Postoperative nausea and vomiting (PONV) and constipation are persistent offenders in this respect.

Practical Analgesic Issues

1. Remember the triad of opiate overdose: *pinpoint pupils, coma, and respiratory depression*. The antidote is naloxone; if you ever need to administer a dose (initial dose = 1 mg iv or im), give it, and then quickly *get help*—it is possible that respiratory depression will return as naloxone is short acting.
2. Note that those patients whose regular analgesic intake must be considered as physiological includes those narcotic addicts whose dependence is being managed by oral methadone. These patients (along with the untreated heroin addict admitted with trauma) can present difficult management problems. Your trust will have a team or nominated individual with responsibility for drug dependency. Their services in concert with the acute pain team will be required in these instances.
3. If you are concerned that an analgesic infusion by whatever route is causing serious mishap, then *STOP*, disconnect the infusion, and get help. *DO NOT* remove the offending catheter unless under the supervision of an anesthetist or the pain team.
4. If there is concern over a patient returned from the operating theater who has had a spinal or epidural anesthetic, note the sensory level of the block achieved in theater. The patient should not return to the ward until this level is fixed or receding. If your examination suggests further proximal progression of the block, summon help immediately.
5. The local anesthetic used in a spinal or epidural anesthetic may have an opiate added to it; this prolongs the analgesic effect,

but note that this can cause *delayed respiratory depression of up to 12 hours*.

6. Be aware of the potential dangers of spinal/epidural anesthesia and thromboprophylaxis. In particular, note that new or progressive neurological deficit developing late in the course of an established epidural infusion or following removal of an epidural catheter may be due to a hematoma causing *spinal cord compression*. This potential catastrophe is discussed in detail in the section Thromboprophylaxis in Chapter 4.

7. A few patients (usually young adults) will develop a spinal headache after an otherwise uneventful administration of spinal anesthetic. This can mimic a subarachnoid hemorrhage, and in the short term the symptoms may be very disabling. Promptly refer such patients to the pain team or responsible anesthetist for confirmation of the diagnosis and further management.

8. Spinal and epidural anesthesia and systemic opiate use are associated with urinary retention, which may be delayed until the postoperative phase. Think of this when reviewing postoperative patients who have not passed urine since returning to the ward.

9. Immediately refer any patient (to the acute pain team or on call anesthetist) with an indwelling pain catheter (epidural or otherwise) who develops signs of local (catheter site) or more generalized sepsis.

10. Know when epidural/spinal or regional anesthesia has been used for a surgical procedure that carries a risk of a *compartment syndrome*. In these patients, the classic symptoms of the syndrome may be absent, disguised, or delayed in the presence of regional or epidural anesthesia. Observe such patients very carefully.

11. Remember also when examining a postoperative limb that successful single-shot major nerve/nerve plexus blocks (e.g., sciatic) can remain anesthetized for up to 24 hours.

12. Interscalene or supraclavicular brachial plexus blocks performed for shoulder and upper limb procedures carry a small incidence of pneumothorax; this needs to be excluded if a recipient experiences postoperative symptoms that might otherwise suggest a pulmonary embolus. The same blocks can also produce an ipsilateral Horner's syndrome; this is self-limiting.

13. As always, respect the physiological status of the elderly and adjust analgesia doses accordingly.

14. If PONV is proving particularly troublesome, make sure while awaiting advice from the pain team that the patient is not

allowed to become significantly dehydrated. Before seeking advice regarding further treatment, review the patient and diagnosis carefully: Are you sure this is analgesia-induced vomiting?

There is no perfect analgesic; best results often result from a balance of different drugs and techniques.

FURTHER READING
See the Thromboprophylaxis section in Chapter 4 and Chapter 12, Compartment Syndrome.

Chapter 7
Dressings, Drains, Plasters, and Tubes

Your patient is likely to return from theatre or arrive from the emergency department with items necessary for their management (Table 7.1). Postoperative instructions should always be the first port of call when doubt exists over how such "accessories" should be managed. There may be departmental protocols for particular procedures—try to understand the rationale for these.

P. Wood et al., *Trauma and Orthopedic Surgery in Clinical Practice*,
DOI: 10.1007/978-1-84800-339-2_7, © Springer-Verlag London Limited 2009

Table 7.1. Postoperative Management of Dressings, Drains, Plasters, and Tubes

Item	Purpose	Care Required
Wound dressings		
There may be different types of dressing used in the same department for the same purpose.	Wound protection and support	Daily inspection of dressing and surrounding areas for evidence of discharge or inflammation
	Absorption of exudate	
	Barrier to infection	Removal and direct inspection of wound if concern exists
Some dressings have special applications (e.g., negative-pressure therapy for large open wounds).	Optimization of wound environment	
Wound packing		
Gauze packing, especially ribbon gauze often soaked in antiseptic	Absorption of exudate	Inspection of area and dressings
Alginate packing also often used	Maintains drainage by keeping wound open	Ensure packing changed regularly, usually at 48-hour intervals
		Failure to change packs increases risk of infective complications, especially toxic shock syndrome
		Deep, packed wounds may require an anesthetic for repacking
Wound drains		
Once a drain has stopped working, it is a potential route for infection.	To remove fluid from a wound	Monitor amount of drainage
Orthopedic wound drains are rarely stitched in.		For fluid balance and calculation of blood loss
Wound drains generally have a radio-opaque marker strip.		To prompt removal when drainage has ceased (usually when sediment appears in the tube)

		Drainage rarely continues beyond 48 hours postop
		Inspection of drain site for signs of infection
		For suction drains, ensure that negative pressure remains
		If incomplete removal suspected, arrange for radiograph to check for retained drain fragment; if so or if drain stuck, will need surgical removal—*inform* seniors immediately
Chest drains	Release of air or fluid (effusion, blood) from the pleural space to ensure reexpansion and effective ventilation of the lung	Do not clamp the tube (risk of tension pneumothorax)
In orthopedics used after trauma (hemo- and pneumothorax, flail chest) and after anterior spinal surgery entering the chest cavity		Do not lift the collecting bottle above the level of the patient's chest (risk of contents siphoning into the chest)
Like wound drains, a nonfunctional chest drain is a conduit for infection and should be removed or replaced.		Duration of use will depend on reason for insertion—*ask* if in doubt
Usually connected to an underwater seal to prevent backflow, but other solutions exist		Regularly check that the drain is "swinging" (i.e., the water level in the underwater seal tube oscillates with respiration); if not, check with seniors as drain may need removal

(Continued)

TABLE 7.1. (Continued)

Item	Purpose	Care Required
		For removal: Cut retaining suture Ask patient to perform a Valsalva maneuver (rehearse before) Remove drain Tie closure suture (usually preinserted) and apply dressing Get chest radiograph
Urethral catheter	Monitors urine output following trauma or major surgery Relief of urinary retention To protect the skin, wounds and dressings from repeated incontinence, especially when the patient is immobile	Observe the fluid balance and act accordingly Remove catheter when no longer needed Use prophylactic antibiotics on catheterization, especially after insertion of orthopedic metal work (risk of bacteremia and infection)
Casts and splints Different materials used, including traditional plaster of Paris and fiberglass Some commercially available splints have complex adjustments; if in doubt, *ask*.	Immobilization of a bone or joint Protection of an inflamed or infected joint Prevention of deformity (e.g., equinus [foot pointing down]) after ankle fracture	Do not ignore pain from beneath a cast; ulceration will eventually stop hurting. Inform a senior immediately so that the cast can be removed or windowed. Oozing from a post-operative wound through a cast may be normal in the immediate post-operative period, but

Support of soft tissues (e.g., after skin graft)

must be monitored. Mark the extent and revisit the patient to check later Attention must be paid to the distal circulation and nerve function: Is the cast too tight? If so, the cast must be split, including all dressings, so that skin is visible. A senior should be informed if this is necessary.

If a plaster splint (backslab) has been opened to check swelling, then it must be rebandaged, and if a fracture may have displaced, a radiograph must be obtained.

FURTHER READING
See Chapter 3, The Ward Round; Chapter 12, Compartment Syndrome; and Chapter 16, the Ill Patient and Medical Emergencies.

Section 3
Special Patient Groups

Chapter 8
The Patient With a Fractured Neck of Femur

A fractured neck of femur (NOF) is the most common reason for admission to an acute orthopedic ward. These patients are usually elderly (>80 years), mostly female (80%), and often have severe comorbidities. Their admissions increase during the winter months, when coincidentally any chronic respiratory disease also tends to worsen. Not uncommonly, they are admitted from care homes or geriatric medical wards while a history of falls is under investigation.

Despite their often poor general medical condition, they are not normally managed in an intensive or high-dependency care setting. Input from elderly care physicians, at an earlier stage, is becoming more common, but this is by no means ubiquitous.

Successful surgical management relies on striking the correct balance between the sometimes conflicting aims of *early surgery*, which is clearly associated with better survival, and optimization of chronic medical conditions.

By contrast, the rare young patient with a fractured NOF also presents a complex, but different, set of priorities as they are typically high-energy injuries associated with other life-threatening trauma and have complications that may cause significant long-term disability. The principles set out in this chapter apply primarily to the elderly patient, but it should be remembered that younger patients will usually require urgent intervention.

SURGICAL CLASSIFICATION OF PROXIMAL FEMUR FRACTURES

Hip fractures are conveniently divided into three groups by the anatomical level of the fracture:

1. *Intracapsular femoral neck fractures* are characterized by risk to the femoral head blood supply with increasing displacement (Figures 8.1, 8.2, 8.3)

P. Wood et al., *Trauma and Orthopedic Surgery in Clinical Practice*,
DOI: 10.1007/978-1-84800-339-2_8, © Springer-Verlag London Limited 2009

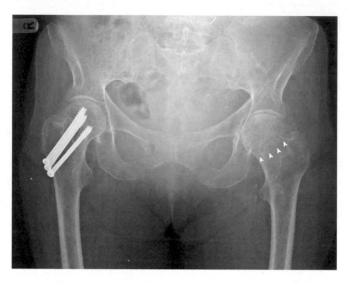

FIGURE 8.1. Minimally displaced intracapsular fractured neck of femur. A new impacted fracture is shown by the arrow on the left. An earlier fracture on the right was treated with cannulated screws.

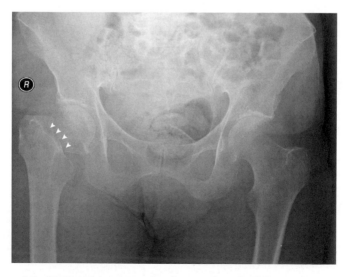

FIGURE 8.2. Displaced intracapsular fractured neck of femur (preoperative). The fracture line is indicated by an arrow on the right femoral neck. Compare the clear profile of the left femoral neck.

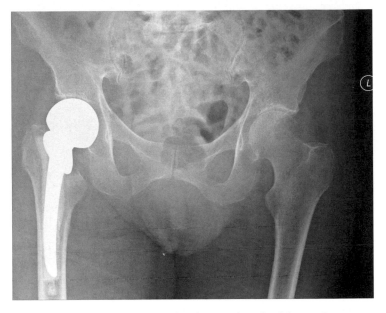

FIGURE 8.3. Displaced intracapsular fractured neck of femur (postoperative). A cemented Thompson hemiarthroplasty has been used to replace the femoral head in the patient shown in Figure 8.2.

2. *Trochanteric fractures* and *basal femoral neck fractures* are extracapsular fractures that lie predominantly in the zone above the lower end of the lesser trochanter (Figures 8.4 and 8.5).
3. *Subtrochanteric fractures* are fractures that predominantly involve the 5 cm of bone below the lesser trochanter. These fractures are much less common than the other two types and are difficult to reduce and surgically complex.

PRINCIPLES OF MANAGEMENT
1. Every attempt should be made to fast track these patients so that early surgery and mobilization can minimize the dangers of prolonged immobility (delays greater than 4 days are associated with a significant increase in mortality). If possible, they should be placed on designated NOF lists to be operated on by suitably experienced staff.
2. The patient's medical condition can frustrate Step 1 but should not prevent early surgery unless it is clear that significant

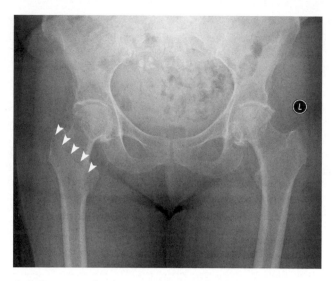

FIGURE 8.4. Extracapsular (intertrochanteric) fractured neck of femur (preoperative. The fracture line is indicated by an arrow on the trochanteric zone of the right femoral neck. This fracture is less displaced than many in this area. Osteoarthritis affects both hip joints.

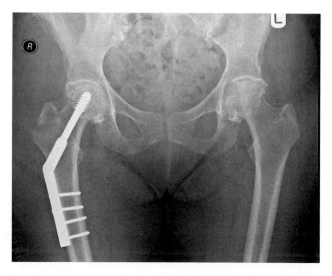

FIGURE 8.5. Extracapsular (intertrochanteric) fractured neck of femur (postoperative). A sliding hip screw, commonly known as a DHS (dynamic hip screw), has been used to stabilize the fracture shown in Figure 8.4.

physiological improvement can be made within a reasonable time frame. This is often a difficult decision, and senior clinical input is essential in dealing with the most ill patients. On occasion, the decision will be made to manage the patient's fracture nonoperatively or with a less-invasive procedure, effectively a palliative fixation.

3. Perioperative care is critical to overall success and will require input from all of the orthopedic support specialties.

4. Even when otherwise fit, the physiology of aging must be respected. Arterial oxygen partial pressure falls with age, as does glomerular filtration rate (GFR). The reduced GFR means that urine output is less and very dependent on a "driving" blood pressure. Blood pressure rises with age such that the normal value for a young adult will equate to hypotension in some elderly patients. The reduction in renal function also means many drugs need to be given in reduced dosage, and any nephrotoxic effects are accentuated.

5. Cognitive function is reduced with aging, and taking elderly patients from their usual environment into a hospital ward often causes disturbances of "awareness," which itself requires careful management (see Chapter 15, The Confused Patient).

YOUR RESPONSIBILITIES

Understand that management of these patients is often complex (Figure 8.6), and they justifiably merit high-priority status in your preparation of patients for the operating theater.

You need to:

1. Clerk the patient as early postadmission as possible. Occasionally, there will be no history available, or you will be reliant on a history given by the patient's caregiver, and details may need to be confirmed with another ward, hospital, or general practitioner. Prescribe analgesia in appropriate doses but be cautious about using nonsteroidal anti-inflammatory drugs (NSAIDs) until it is clear that there are no renal problems. Thromboembolic prophylaxis should be prescribed according to your departmental policy; these patients are at high risk of venous thromboembolism.

2. Routine blood checks should include a complete blood count (CBC) and analysis of urea and electrolytes. A 12-lead electrocardiogram (ECG) is mandatory, as is a chest X-ray. Severe chest disease will also require evaluation of arterial blood gases.

3. Be proactive in following up the results from Step 2.

4. Postoperatively review these patients frequently. Postoperative chest infection, confusion, and problems with fluid management are not unusual.

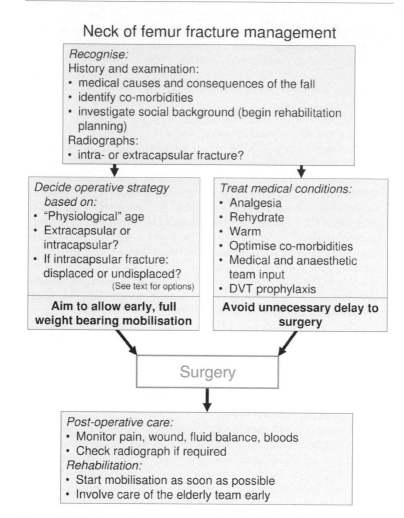

Figure 8.6. Pathway for management of neck-of-femur fractures in elderly patients. Actions with a dark grey background could be managed by a junior member of the team, but light grey and grey actions will require senior input.

Specific Issues

1. Patients with chronic pulmonary obstructive pulmonary disease (COPD): Ensure that the chest X-ray and blood gases are available and get an early anesthetic opinion in respect to fitness for surgery.

2. Atrial fibrillation: If this is unstable (causing hypotension or heart rate persistently > 100 beats per minute), it poses real problems for anesthesia. It may be related to a chest infection or chronic cardiac pathology. Check the serum potassium and inform the anesthetist or orthopedic physician for guidance. A related issue is patients on warfarin (see Chapter 4, Thromboprophylaxis section).

3. If the patient is clearly in acute on chronic heart failure, then surgery will most certainly be delayed; get an urgent medical opinion.

4. If the patient has a pacemaker, follow the guidance given in Chapter 4, Preparing Patients for Operation.

5. Anemic patients: Extracapsular fractures in particular can bleed heavily. Nearly all NOF patients will require a preoperative hemolytic group-andsave procedure as a minimum, and some will require preoperative transfusion. If you are unsure, *ask* but do note that the current trend in transfusion medicine that permits young surgical patients to maintain a low hemoglobin *is not* an appropriate strategy for these patients.

6. Electrolyte disturbances: Pay particular attention to the serum potassium. It needs to be in the normal range before surgery. If the patient's urea is elevated from dehydration, then commence an intravenous infusion *BUT DO NOT* use 5% dextrose. Prolonged infusion of water will cause hyponatremia, which will also delay operation and may in itself prove fatal. The "3 L a day" of the young *is not* an appropriate prescription for an underweight, frail, elderly female, in whom it is easy to precipitate acute left ventricular failure.

7. Consent: A significant proportion of the patients will have dementia or a confusional state that cannot be improved before surgery is needed. Adhere to the principles outlined in Chapters 4 on consent. It is particularly important to communicate effectively with the patient's relatives, who may be unaware how a fractured NOF is a life- and mobility-threatening injury.

At times, these patients will severely test your clinical acumen. It is important to remember that even when managed in an exemplary fashion, the 1 year mortaility is 33%.

FURTHER READING

See Chapter 4, Preparing Patients for Operation, Parts I and II; Chapter 5, Intravenous Fluids and Electrolytes; and all chapters in Section 4, Problems and Complications: The Patient.

Chapter 9
Rheumatoid Arthritis

Patients suffering from rheumatoid arthritis present a constant orthopedic workload, especially in hand units. These patients have multisystem problems that can influence their perioperative course. You need to be mindful of the items discussed in this chapter.

GENERAL CONSIDERATIONS

These patients are often elderly, sometimes severely disabled, and often the recipients of many surgical procedures. They are often frail, with thin skin that is prone to ulceration. This situation is often made worse by long-term dependence on steroids. Their joint pathology is generalized and includes the cervical spine and temporomandibular joint. Severe cases may have a marked flexion deformity of their neck. Aside from joint and soft tissue issues, they can also present with chronic anemia, restrictive lung disease, and renal impairment from amyloid or drug therapy. Their immobility will occasionally disguise the presence of ischemic heart disease or cardiac conduction defects. The combination of drugs (steroids, immunosuppressants, antacids) and anemia make postoperative infection more likely.

PREPARATION FOR SURGERY

It is important that you:

1. Discuss any special radiological requirements with your seniors. The anesthetist may request cervical spine views. These should not be ordered as a routine until the anesthetist has had the opportunity to visit the patient. The anesthetist's decision regarding whether these are required will be based on a functional assessment of the patient's airway and inquiry about any previous anesthesia. If your own clerking reveals previous operative issues, then make sure the relevant old notes are available or have been requested.

P. Wood et al., *Trauma and Orthopedic Surgery in Clinical Practice*,
DOI: 10.1007/978-1-84800-339-2_9, © Springer-Verlag London Limited 2009

2. When pulmonary function is affected, a chest X-ray or arterial blood gases may be needed. On rare occasions, formal lung function tests (if not performed previously) may be necessary. If you suspect that this could be the case, inform the responsible anesthetist at the earliest opportunity. If suspicious of ischemic heart disease, ensure a 12-lead electrocardiogram (ECG) is available.

3. Discuss with the operating surgeon estimated blood loss. If the patient is anemic, then preoperative cross matching of blood may become necessary.

4. If it is thought important to prevent preoperative dehydration, then take care with the cannula placement and dressing. Sites may be limited, and the combination of thin skin and fragile veins often leads to failure.

POSTOPERATIVE CARE

Important considerations here include:

1. Increased doses of steroids may be necessary for a varying period depending on the nature of the surgery. Normally, these can be given orally *but* be prepared to switch to the intravenous route if nausea or vomiting prevents oral absorption.

2. Ask about and watch carefully for any upper gastrointestinal symptoms that suggest the possibility of hemorrhage. This may result from increased perioperative use of nonsteroidal anti-inflammatory analgesics or steroids plus the effects of routine thromboprophylaxis. If not already prescribed, review the necessity for gastric protection (e.g., with ranitidine, omeprazole, or antacids).

3. Following prolonged or significant surgical procedures, check the postoperative hemoglobin, urea, and electrolyte values.

4. Be alert to the clinical and laboratory signs/markers of postoperative infection.

5. Examine the patient's dependent areas. This is particularly important when surgery has been prolonged or carried out under a regional block (often the case in rheumatoid patients).

> Rheumatoid arthritis is a multisystem disorder—beware of treatment-related immunosuppression.

FURTHER READING

See Chapter 4's section, Concurrent Medication.

Chapter 10
Hemophilia

BACKGROUND

The United Kingdom has some 6,000 registered hemophiliacs; 90% of these will suffer from hemophilia A and are deficient in factor 8. The reminder have von Willebrand's disease, a deficiency of factor 9. The severity of hemophilia A is classed according to base levels of factor 8 (normal range = 50–150 IU/dL). Patients with the severe form (factor level < 1 IU/dL) require regular prophylactic treatment to prevent disabling bleeding into joints and soft tissues.

Prior to 1985, the process used to prepare plasma concentrates were not virucidal; as a consequence, the United Kingdom hemophiliac population contains some 360 HIV-positive patients and 5,000 with hepatitis B or C. Many of the latter group have developed progressive liver disease. The situation is complicated still further by the 30% of patients who develop inhibitors (antibodies) to their missing factor.

The complexity of their condition means that care is undertaken in multidisciplinary centers headed by hematologists and their specialist nurses. Arrangements are in place for 24-hour care so that acute episodes can be correctly managed.

You should appreciate that most of these patients are highly informed about their condition and in particular how to respond to an acute crisis (which a patient will often self-manage at home).

ORTHOPEDIC PRESENTATION

Hemophiliac patients may present acutely because of acute joint or muscle hematoma (including a risk of compartment syndrome). Elective surgery includes:

1. Complications of soft tissue hemorrhage, including pseudotumors (encapsulated hematomas following repeated bleeding into soft tissues or bone)

P. Wood et al., *Trauma and Orthopedic Surgery in Clinical Practice*,
DOI: 10.1007/978-1-84800-339-2_10, © Springer-Verlag London Limited 2009

2. Correction of joint contractures: Tendon procedures and osteotomy
3. Synovectomy for chronic synovitis
4. Arthrodesis or joint replacement (especially of the knee)

There no such thing as minor surgery in a hemophiliac, and any orthopedic surgeon operating on these patients will have a specialized interest in this field.

PREOPERATIVE PREPARATION

Talk to people. The patient's admission will be known to the hemophilia team, whose nurses can be expected to organize the presurgery factor 8 assay and the subsequent dosing and administration of concentrate. You must communicate with this team to find out what (if any) areas of this responsibility they wish you to take on. If the hematology nurses prescribe, then check their arithmetic (factor units per kilogram) for yourself.

Confirm that theaters and the anesthetists have been informed by the operating surgeon of this patient and the proposed nature and time of surgery.

Factor Levels

For surgery, 50 units/kg of factor 8 will be given intravenously to produce levels of 100% of normal. The half-life of factor 8 is approximately 24 hours, so postoperatively some 25 units/kg will be administered every 8–12 hours for around 5–7 days. Thereafter, levels of 30–50% of normal should be sufficient up to the time of patient discharge.

Patients with inhibitors will require specialized factor products and are especially prone to postoperative complications.

POSTOPERATIVE CARE

You should:

1. Perform investigations and assays as requested by the hemophilia and theater teams. The postoperative hemoglobin value will be particularly important if transfusion or blood salvage techniques were needed.
2. Again, cross-check all elective factor concentrate prescriptions with the hematology nurses. If asked by the hemophilia team to prescribe an unfamiliar preparation or additional concentrate as an emergency (e.g., postoperative bleeding), get a colleague to check any math required.

3. *Do not* permit use of the intramuscular route and *do not* prescribe any anticoagulants or drugs (aspirin, nonsteroidal anti-inflammatory drugs [NSAIDs]), which may cause gastrointestinal bleeding. Consequently, pain control can be difficult, and you may need advice from the pain control team.

4. Think before undertaking or requesting otherwise routine procedures such as a dressing or cast change. To permit such activity and to allow physiotherapy, the factor 8 level will need to be at least 30% of normal.

5. In addition to routine clinical signs, keep a close check on wounds, dressings, and drains for signs of bleeding. Factor 8 is a cofactor (with factor 10) in producing a stable clot at the end of the coagulation cascade. Hemophilia is therefore defined by a failure of clot integrity, and late bleeding is a concern. Another problem from bleeding is a compartment syndrome, which is a particular risk for patients with inhibitors.

6. Think always about the possibility of infection, another common complication made worse still in the presence of HIV immunosuppression.

> Perioperative preparation for hemophiliacs relies on effective communication and teamwork.

FURTHER READING
See Chapter 11, Infection and Immunocompromise, and Chapter 12, Compartment Syndrome.

Section 4

Problems and Complications:
The Patient

Chapter 11
Infection and Immunocompromise

The presence of infection or altered immunity may seriously complicate the management of orthopedic patients, especially when a prosthesis is in place. The patient may acquire the infection during hospitalization, or it may (as an acute or chronic problem, e.g., osteomyelitis, infected joint replacement) be the reason for either emergency or elective admission.

DEFINITIONS

Bacteremia: The entry of organisms into the bloodstream. This process may be transient or sustained and may or may not be limited by the patient's immune response or the effect of prophylactic antibiotics.

Infection: The colonization of previously healthy tissue or wounds by microbiological organisms.

Sepsis: The combination of infection and a systemic inflammatory response syndrome (SIRS).

Septic shock: Sepsis in association with hypotension as a result of sustained SIRS.

The relationship between these definitions and the potential for progression to multiple organ failure is shown in Figure 11.1.

VULNERABILITY TO INFECTION

Medical conditions that increase the risk of acquiring hospital infection are not uncommon in orthopedic patients and include:

1. Immunosuppression from chronic medical problems, previous trauma, or existing infection (e.g., chronic obstructive pulmonary disease [COPD], postsplenectomy patients, HIV infection)
2. Drug-induced immunosuppression, including steroids (e.g., in rheumatoid arthritis and posttransplant patients)
3. Poor nutritional status (the elderly, after prolonged hospitalization), alcohol and substance abuse

P. Wood et al., *Trauma and Orthopedic Surgery in Clinical Practice*,
DOI: 10.1007/978-1-84800-339-2_11, © Springer-Verlag London Limited 2009

4. Cigarette smoking
5. Malignancy
6. Old age

Some patients will have more than one condition, but following injury or surgery, all are at risk of infection because of

1. Postoperative respiratory complications
2. Delayed and poor wound healing
3. Exacerbation or progression of their preexisting pathology

HISTORY AND EXAMINATION

In the presence of actual or suspected infection, preexisting risk factors may be offered by both the patient and previous medical records. Signs of infection or altered immunity may include pyrexia, non-trauma-related tachypnea or tachycardia, lymphadenopathy, splenomegaly, cellulitis, and phlebitis. Infected wounds not only may smell but also are often disproportionately painful. Infected joints are locally associated with restriction of movement, swelling, tense overlying skin, and again severe pain.

LABORATORY AND RADIOLOGICAL INVESTIGATION OF INFECTION

Supporting or confirmatory evidence may follow from hematology: anemia, abnormal white cell count (classically neutrophil leukocytosis), thrombocytopenia, raised erythrocyte sedimentation rate (ESR), and an elevated C-reactive protein (CRP) level.

Liver function tests may be abnormal in patients with hepatitis.

Tissue/wound, blood, urine, sputum and stool cultures may also be necessary.

Radiological imaging will be determined by the clinical problem, but usually plain X-rays will be performed before specialized techniques.

POSTOPERATIVE INFECTION

Postoperative infection may be localized to the site of surgery, or if the patient is unwell, then the systemic effects of infection may be accelerating (Figure 11.1).

Sepsis

The intravascular dissemination of bacteria and their toxic products is *bacteremia*; if the systemic response to the bacteremia causes circulatory dysfunction, then the patient is *septic* (Figure 11.1).

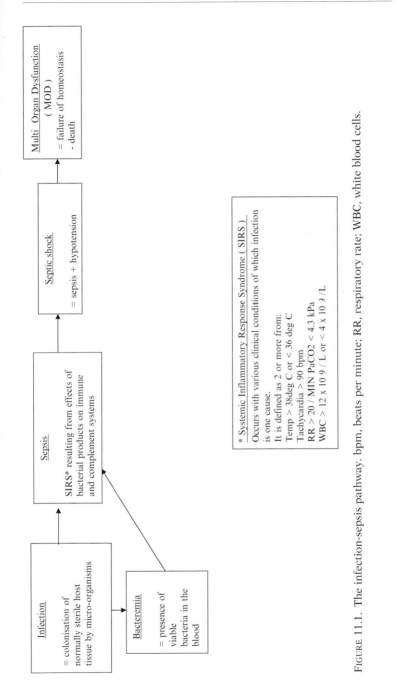

FIGURE 11.1. The infection-sepsis pathway. bpm, beats per minute; RR, respiratory rate; WBC, white blood cells.

The essential pathophysiology is reduced tissue perfusion; the clinical signs and symptoms reflect this and include confusion, tachypnea, tachycardia, systolic hypotension, and poor urine output. The patient may be pyrexial, and occasionally nonspecific skin rashes or hemorrhages may be found.

Laboratory investigations may reveal any of the features listed, and coagulopathy is also a feature in severe cases. Note that in the presence of immunosuppression or chemotherapy, the white cell count be may be normal or low. Blood and wound cultures may reveal the offending organism, but these and all of the stated signs, symptoms, and other investigations may be deceptive if the patient is already receiving antibiotics.

Having assessed the patients general condition, a head-to-toe inspection is required, concentrating on wounds and then all "foreign material" must be inspected, including dressings, pins, catheters, drains, and the like.

If the patients is sick, then the *ABC* approach (see Chapter 16, The Ill Patient and Medical Emergencies) must be rigorously followed, and *early* contact with the intensive care unit (ICU) team is necessary. *Microbiological advice is mandatory as prompt antimicrobial treatment is essential.* The microbiologists will recommend an empirical prescription that will take account of the patient's medical history, the likely source (or sources) of the infection, local flora (and antimicrobial sensitivities), and any current antibiotic treatment.

Depending on the perceived origin of the sepsis, the patient may need to return to the operating theater.

Sepsis can initially present covertly, but the patient can go from a state of minimal physiological upset to death very quickly from multiorgan failure secondary to hypotension. You should always suspect this diagnosis in any postoperative patient who becomes "generally" unwell, and such cases mandate an urgent senior review.

Health Care-Associated Infection

Each year in the United Kingdom, some 9% of in-patients (100,000) acquire infection as a consequence of their hospitalization; 11% of these are postoperative wound infections. Health care-associated infections (HCAIs) include those caused by methicillin-resistant *Staphylococcus aureus* (MRSA) and *Clostridium difficile* (*C. diff*).

Notes on Methicillin-Resistant Staphylococcus aureus and Clostridium difficile Infections

Patients and their relatives understandably fear the possibility of catching one of the "superbugs." You must expect to be questioned by people whose emotions over this subject will range from the concerned to the overtly hostile. Some background information is included here (Table 11.1), but it is not unusual to be asked directly regarding the incidence in your unit. The reporting of MRSA bacteremia and *C. diff* infections is a mandatory requirement, and data are published quarterly. In the United Kingdom, your hospital's latest figures can be viewed at the Health Protection Agency (HPA) site (see Bibliography at the end of this book).

Preventing Iatrogenic Infection

It is no accident that this missive on preventing iatrogenic infection appears next to the notes on MRSA and *C. diff*.

Be responsible: This means wash your hands between patients, use alcohol rubs freely (particularly on traveling between wards), and dress appropriately (gown, gloves, etc.) when carrying out patient procedures.

If in doubt over sterile procedure, consult the nursing staff.

PRINCIPLES OF MANAGING INFECTED OR IMMUNOCOMPROMISED PATIENTS

The essential rules for managing infected or immunocompromised patients are as follows:

1. *Constantly be alert to the ease with which localized infection can become systemic sepsis and septicemic shock, a condition that can be rapidly fatal.* (This message is so important its recognition and management are repeated in Chapter 15, The Ill Patient and Medical Emergencies).
2. Establish previous tetanus immunity; immunize or boost as necessary.
3. Ensure asplenic patients have had, or will receive, pneumococcal vaccine (specific advice available in the British National Formulary).
4. Do not vaccinate chemotherapy patients without specialist advice.
5. Take all necessary samples (e.g., biopsy, joint aspiration) for microbiology before giving prophylactic antibiotics. When completing specimen forms, ensure that the medical history is sufficient to ensure proper investigation by the laboratory.

TABLE 11.1. Methicillin-Resistant *Staphylococcus aureus* (MRSA) and *Clostridium difficile*

	MRSA	C. difficile
Background	High incidence (1:3) of asymptomatic carriers permits hospital patient colonization with or without infection	Infection results from gut overgrowth of normal commensal (3% of adults) due to antibiotic therapy. The *C. diff* toxin is detected in stool of infected patient.
Cofactors	1. Ease with which *S. aureus* can enter body via wounds, catheters, cannulae, etc. 2. Propensity for antibiotic resistance when exposed to sicker patients receiving multiple or prolonged antimicrobial treatments 3. Associated with item 2 is a natural increase in infection rates in hospitals performing specialized and complex surgery	1. Prophylactic use of broad-spectrum antibiotics in orthopedics 2. Increasing age (over 80% of cases occur in patients aged 65 or over)
Clinical presentation	Either by detection of carriers or following investigation of wound/prosthesis infection or bacteremia	Mild diarrhea to severe hemorrhagic colitis
Treatment	1. Eradication in asymptomatic carriers with antiseptics. Some units will have protocols for planned elective surgery. 2. Prolonged and often difficult (intravenous) therapy with antibiotics as determined by sensitivity.	Oral metronidazole 400 mg three times a day or oral vancomycin 125 mg three times a day Inadequate evidence for routine use of probiotics Potentially fatal in the old (20%).
Outcome	Variable; has a definite mortality. Recovered patients will require a negative screen before any hospital readmission.	Some patients will become chronic carriers, but this should not delay discharge to home or residential care once patient has been symptom free for 48 hours. There is a 20–30% relapse rate.

6. When taking blood cultures, inoculate the anaerobic bottle first.

7. Invasive procedures such as urinary catheterization are associated with bacteremia, and intravenous antibiotic cover must be given if the patient has "metal work" in situ.

8. Involve specialist help as necessary, particularly in respect of the ongoing management of any underlying chronic condition or the need for specialized products (e.g., irradiated blood products).

9. Be prepared to measure and adjust blood levels of therapeutic agents according to microbiology advice.

10. Consider the need for increased steroid dosage postinjury or postsurgery.

11. Always review the serial trend when examining laboratory markers of infection.

12. Reduce the risk to other patients. Establish a liaison with nursing colleagues to ensure necessary precautions are taken in the management and placement of patients in the operating theater and the wards. This will include annotating the theater list when MRSA-infected patients are due for surgery.

THE RISK TO YOURSELF

The risk to yourself is the possibility of acquiring infection through direct contact with body fluids, inhalation, or inoculation, usually needle-stick injury. Trauma patients frequently present from complicated medical and social backgrounds. Infections such as hepatitis B and HIV are not uncommon. The real risk is that which is not known; this is minimized by preparation and adherence to some simple rules and common sense.

1. For invasive and exposure-prone procedures wear appropriate protective clothing at all times, especially gloves.

2. Respect and adhere to local infection control and occupational health policies, particularly with respect to hepatitis B.

3. Take responsibility for cross infection; we say again, wash your hands between patients and use skin scrubs as supplied.

4. In the unlikely event of a needle-stick injury, know and comply with the local occupational health policies for investigation and treatment.

With postoperative wound infection and a sick patient—think sepsis.

FURTHER READING
See Chapter 3, The Ward Round; Chapter 7, Dressings, Drains, Plasters, and Tubes; and Chapter 16, The Ill Patient and Medical Emergencies.

Chapter 12
Compartment Syndrome

THE PROBLEM

Compartment syndrome occurs when swollen muscles within an unyielding envelope become ischemic as the capillary closing pressure is exceeded. The envelope in question typically consists of the *fascia* and *bone* surrounding the muscle, but skin and external restrictions such as *encircling dressings* and *plaster splints* may contribute to the situation. The consequences for a patient may be disastrous.

In the acute situation, severe pain results, and in the long term, if untreated, muscle necrosis results in fibrosis and consequent stiffness—the classical Volkmann's ischemic contracture.

Muscle can tolerate only 4 hours of ischemia before irreversible changes occur. Failure to recognize compartment syndrome is a potent source of litigation.

CAUSES

Any cause of swelling can result in compartment syndrome if this occurs within a muscle compartment. The most common causes seen in trauma and orthopedic practice are:

- Associated with fractures and dislocations, either acutely or after surgery on the injury
- Following reperfusion of a limb when there has been prolonged ischemia
- As a consequence of vessel injury and bleeding into a compartment

It is worth remembering that *any* fracture, open or closed, may result in a compartment syndrome.

Some injuries do carry a more worrisome reputation. The classic example is a closed tibial shaft fracture, but supracondylar fracture of the humerus, crush injuries, foot fractures, and dislocations are of concern.

P. Wood et al., *Trauma and Orthopedic Surgery in Clinical Practice*,
DOI: 10.1007/978-1-84800-339-2_12, © Springer-Verlag London Limited 2009

PREVENTION

Standard fracture care will help to reduce the consequences of muscle swelling:

- Admission and careful observation of all patients with crush injuries, lower-limb long-bone fractures, and any injury associated with significant swelling and pain
- Elevation of the affected part to heart level
- Avoidance of tight encircling dressings
- Use of splintage that is easily removed (e.g., plaster backslab, split cast)
- Continuous monitoring of compartment pressures, if appropriate (see the next section).

RECOGNITION

The diagnosis of compartment syndrome is *clinical*. In some circumstances, this will need to be supported by measurement of compartment pressures.

The cardinal symptom of compartment syndrome is *severe pain*, out of proportion to the injury. Seeking other features of ischemia—pallor, paresthesia, loss of pulses, and paralysis—is not helpful in diagnosis as they are either absent or often delayed beyond the time at which irreversible muscle damage occurs.

One helpful clinical sign is the *increase in pain that occurs on passive stretch of a muscle.*

The following points are helpful:

- Pain from fractures typically improves with splintage: *Beware the injury with increased pain after splintage.*
- The pain of compartment syndrome is so severe that one might feel the patient is complaining excessively or seeking opiate analgesia inappropriately. It is important to resist this temptation and be suspicious of compartment syndrome.
- A patient with a compartment syndrome will often appear extremely distracted and unable to conduct a normal conversation.
- Beware the injury in a patient with altered level of consciousness, including drug or alcohol intoxication, or altered perception of pain, such as neuropathy or spinal cord injury.
- In the postoperative patient, beware of compartment syndrome after prolonged tourniquet use or if local anesthetic blocks, spinal anesthesia, or epidural anesthesia have been used.

Compartment syndrome management

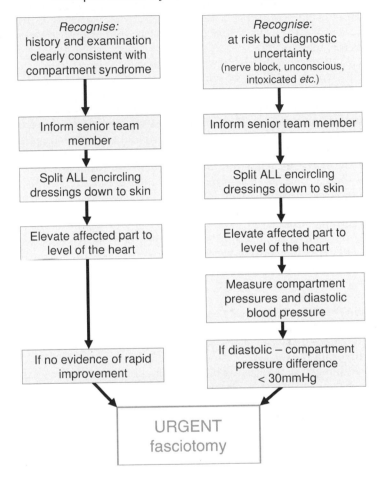

FIGURE 12.1. Pathway for management of compartment syndrome in trauma patients. Actions with a dark grey background could be managed by a junior member of the team, but light grey and grey actions will require senior input.

A clear clinical presentation of compartment syndrome requires no further investigation to confirm diagnosis as this will only delay the necessarily urgent treatment.

If the diagnosis is doubtful, for example, if a local anesthetic block has been used, then compartment pressure measurement can be used for confirmation. Although it is possible to construct a simple device for such measurements from ward equipment, it is more usual now to use a dedicated electronic device or a pressure sensor such as used for continuous arterial or central venous pressure monitoring.

While you would not be expected to set up and conduct such monitoring yourself, it is sensible to know where such a kit is located so that it can be easily found in an emergency.

The level at which a compartment pressure is regarded as diagnostic of compartment syndrome is somewhat variable from one surgeon to the next; a commonly used definition is to regard a compartment syndrome to be present when the difference between the compartment pressure and the patient's diastolic pressure is less than 30 mm Hg. It is important to measure *all compartments in the suspected part* (e.g., in four compartments in the leg) as only one compartment may be affected and to repeat measurements if concern persists.

Continuous monitoring may be justified in patients with altered conscious level or sensation.

The pathway to management of the syndrome is presented in Fig. 12.1.

TREATMENT

Once a compartment syndrome is suspected, any dressings, including casts or backslabs, should be opened, splitting all layers so that skin is exposed.

Although the underlying bone will no longer be supported, this is a secondary concern compared to the effects of compartment syndrome.

The affected part should be elevated to heart level to optimize circulation.

Once an *immediate senior review* has confirmed the diagnosis, urgent surgical management is needed. This will involve surgical release of the fascial envelope of the compartments (termed a *fasciotomy*). In the leg, this is usually accomplished through two long incisions, one medial and one lateral. If there is an unstabilized fracture, this should be stabilized after the compartment release. Fasciotomy wounds are left open after release to avoid recurrence.

After the surgery, pain usually falls quite quickly, but the size of the fasciotomy wounds and bulging of the underlying muscle will often preclude later direct closure so that a delayed split skin graft may be necessary.

If the problem is spotted and treated promptly, then functional limitation is unlikely, but scars may be unsightly, and fractures in association with a compartment syndrome may heal more slowly and may become infected as the fasciotomy effectively converts a closed into an open fracture.

In those limbs at risk, progressively increasing pain is a compartment syndrome until proved otherwise.

FURTHER READING
See Chapter 6, Analgesia.

Chapter 13
Deep Venous Thrombosis and Pulmonary Embolism

Orthopedic patients are at particular risk of thromboembolic disease (see the discussion in Chapter 4's Thromboprophylaxis section). There is a wealth of literature in leading medical journals concerning the stratification of risk and accuracy of diagnostic tests in thromboembolic disease, but despite this some orthopedic patients will suffer a deep venous thrombosis (DVT).

The origin of 90% of venous thrombi is in the lower extremities. Up to 50% of these will embolize as pulmonary emboli (PE), with an overall estimated mortality of 6–15%. Pulmonary embolism is the most common postmortem finding after in-hospital cardiac arrest.

Your role in the orthopedic ward is to understand the increased risk of these conditions in this patient group and ensure that correct precautions have been taken (again, see Thromboprophylaxis in Chapter 4). You should be alert to the relevant signs and symptoms and direct the attention of your seniors to any individual patient giving cause for concern.

DEEP VENOUS THROMBOSIS

Diagnosis
The possibility of a DVT must be entertained when examining a "symptomatic lower limb." The usual complaints are of pain or swelling. Clinical examination is unreliable, but you should attempt to exclude other causes, including cellulitis, hematoma, refracture, acute arterial ischemia, and compartment syndrome. If the problem is bilateral, congestive cardiac failure is a possibility.

The diagnosis is best confirmed by duplex ultrasound, which requires a radiologist. Ultrasound is best for proximal thrombosis, less so for calf vein thrombosis, and on occasion the radiologists will perform computerized tomographic (CT) venography.

P. Wood et al., *Trauma and Orthopedic Surgery in Clinical Practice*,
DOI: 10.1007/978-1-84800-339-2_13, © Springer-Verlag London Limited 2009

Treatment

Treatment has been simplified by the introduction of low molecular weight heparins (LMWHs), which have the advantage of being given subcutaneously once daily (long half-life), with predictable effect and no need to monitor the activated partial thromboplastin time (APPT). Contemporaneous with the administration of heparin, oral anticoagulation is commenced with warfarin. This will be continued subsequently as an outpatient with the aim of maintaining an international normalized ratio (INR) of 2.5.

Your unit should have a protocol for routine anticoagulation. The problem is with the definition of what is routine. The advice of the hematologist should always be sought in difficult cases, such as patients who are facing further surgery because of staged procedures or the patient who has a recurrent history of thromboembolism.

PULMONARY EMBOLUS

The presentation of pulmonary embolism (PE) will range from the cheerful patient who adds as an aside on the ward round, "Strange, I feel a little breathless today, doctor," to the asymptomatic individual who collapses in cardiorespiratory arrest.

Dyspnea, pleuritic pain, and *hemoptysis* are the most frequent symptoms; any such complaints must be taken seriously.

Inquire regarding the time of onset of symptoms and ask specifically about pleuritic pain and hemoptysis. Study the observations chart; *a rise in respiratory rate may be the only clue, and a respiratory rate above 20 will be found in around 70% of patients.* Some 30% of patients will have associated tachycardia.

Look for the potential origin of an embolus; examine the legs as for DVT. Clinical examination of the chest may reveal the presence of a pleural rub or crepitations secondary to infarction.

Get a plain chest X-ray (CXR; pneumothorax needs to be excluded) and 12-lead electrocardiogram (ECG). The ECG may well appear normal (in particular, do not expect to find the classic S1 Q3 T3 pattern; nonspecific ST/T wave changes are more likely). It may of course also reveal an alternative diagnosis.

Take an arterial blood gas on air; both the PaO_2 and $PaCO_2$ will typically be *low*.

The measurement of D-dimer (a product of fibrin formed in the thrombotic process) in an inpatient orthopedic ward is not required. Elevated levels are seen in various acute inflammatory conditions, and while a negative result in a patient at low risk excludes PE, a positive result (however raised) does not make the diagnosis more likely in high-risk orthopedic patients.

Be prepared to discuss the case with the radiologist and physicians, particularly if the patient has any previous cardiac or respiratory history. Computerized tomographic pulmonary angiography (CPTA) is now regarded as the definitive and first-line investigation, although it is possible that a ventilation/perfusion (V/Q) scan will be performed in certain cases.

Table 13.1 provides the key features of PEs.

TABLE 13.1. Pulmonary Embolism (PE): Key Features

Your Responsibility[a]	
Patient: Symptoms and signs	Dyspnea, ± tachypnea, ± pleuritic chest pain (not positional), ± hemoptysis; chest wall pain unrelated to trauma
	↑ RR (>20 breaths per minute = significant), tachycardia, pleural rub, crepitations, wheeze (new onset), pyrexia
Initial investigations	CXR: Frequently initially normal, possible linear atelectasis and later more extensive collapse/consolidation; pleural effusion + raised hemidiaphragm also late signs
	ECG: sinus rhythm/sinus tachycardia, AF, evidence of right heart strain (S_1 Q_3 T_3 pattern or RBBB); most frequently nonspecific ST segment changes
	Arterial blood gases: ↓ PaO_2, ↓ $PaCO_2$
Middle- or Senior-Grade Review[b]	
Further investigations	Consideration of alternative diagnosis D-dimer test (low-risk patients only)
Senior-Level Decisions	
Radiology + hematology opinion	Immediate LMWH→CPTA
Definitive treatment	Oral warfarin once diagnosis confirmed

AF, atrial fibrillation; CPTA, computerized tomographic pulmonary angiography; CXR, chest X-ray; LMWH, low molecular weight heparin; RBBB, right bundle branch block; RR, respiratory rate.

[a] These are your responsibility – if there is any suspicion of PE, investigate as shown and *immediately* refer for a more senior orthopedic opinion.

[b] Middle- or senior-grade review is needed to confirm or otherwise.

[c] Decisions on need for imaging and immediate/long-term treatment are to be made at the senior level.

The Sick Patient With a Pulmonary Embolism

Around 15% of patients will present with syncope or collapse with no prodromal symptoms. Some of these patients will clearly be extremely ill, and resuscitation is necessary in tandem with diagnosis. (See chapter 16, The ill patient).

A massive embolus may be diagnosed with bedside echocardiography.

Treatment of Pulmonary Embolism

Subcutaneous LMWH should be given before any radiological studies. If the patient is unwell, then intravenous unfractionated heparin is an alternative; individual management should be discussed with a hematologist. The patient should be given oxygen during transport to the radiology department as this will help to minimize hypoxic pulmonary vasoconstriction. Oral anticoagulation (target INR is the same as for DVT) should await diagnostic confirmation.

The small group of very ill patients with a massive embolus will require thrombolysis or assessment for surgical intervention. Their treatment will be prescribed and supervised in the high-dependency unit or intensive care unit.

> If dyspnea/tachypnea or hemoptysis occur with or without pleuritic chest pain, the diagnosis is pulmonary embolism until proven otherwise.

FURTHER READING

In Chapter 4, see the Thromboprophylaxis section; also see Chapter 16, The Ill Patient and Medical Emergencies.

Chapter 14
Fat Embolism

Fat embolism results from systemic embolization of fat from disrupted marrow or adipose tissue. Arterial-venous shunting allows dispersion throughout the vascular system, while biochemical modification of the fat may also contribute to any subsequent clinical effects.

Some authorities consider fat embolism to be a universal effect of long-bone fracture, and many cases are clinically silent. Clinical manifestations usually present within 24–72 hours postinjury and positively correlate with the severity of injury; on occasions, the condition be life threatening.

It may occur during orthopedic surgery and is also associated with pancreatitis following abdominal trauma.

PRESENTATION

A textbook presentation is unlikely, but fat embolism may be associated with any of the following and classically the first three:

1. *Respiratory distress:* The patient may complain of dyspnea, and the only abnormal physical finding is tachypnea. Oximetry and blood gas analysis will reveal reduced oxygenation, which may become progressive. Rarely, the presentation may be one of catastrophic cardiorespiratory collapse, as with a massive pulmonary embolism.
2. *Neurological:* This can occur directly from cerebral emboli or indirectly secondary to hypoxia. Presenting features include mild confusion to coma. Localizing neurological deficits may occur.
3. *Skin:* Skin involvement is revealed as a petechial rash over the upper half of the body.
4. *Eyes:* Conjunctival petechiae and rarely fundoscopy may display retinal vessel emboli.
5. *Renal:* There may be reduced urine output.

P. Wood et al., *Trauma and Orthopedic Surgery in Clinical Practice*,
DOI: 10.1007/978-1-84800-339-2_14, © Springer-Verlag London Limited 2009

CONFIRMING THE DIAGNOSIS

There is no absolute confirmatory test; the diagnosis is made clinically. A high index of suspicion should apply to all long-bone (especially femur) and pelvic fracture patients who suffer any form of respiratory compromise.

Examine the patient and the patient's observations chart. Sometimes, the only abnormal finding will be a persistent and otherwise unexplained tachypnea or tachycardia, possibly associated with pyrexia.

Chest auscultation may reveal crepitations. A chest X-ray (CXR) is necessary to exclude other causes of hypoxia; by itself, significant fat embolism may be revealed by a "snowstorm" appearance.

Arterial blood gases will quantify the degree of hypoxia, and an electrocardiogram (ECG) should be obtained.

Venous blood sampling may reveal anemia, thrombocytopenia, a raised erythrocyte sedimentation rate (ESR), and rarely hypo–calcemia.

If the presentation is neurological, then computerized tomographic (CT) imaging may be necessary to exclude other pathologies.

TREATMENT

Treatment is supportive (i.e., oxygen). No specific therapy exists either to prevent ongoing embolization (other than fracture stabilization) or to reverse the effects already present. It is also important to ensure that the patient is not hypovolemic. and that thromboprophylaxis is in place.

If hypoxia or oliguria are severe or there is significant neurological deficit, then help must be sought from the intensive care team.

Fat embolism is an important differential clinical diagnosis when there are postoperative respiratory problems.

FURTHER READING

See Chapter 12, Deep Venous Thrombosis and Pulmonary Embolism, and Chapter 16, The Ill Patient and Medical Emergencies,.

Chapter 15
The Confused Patient

On the orthopedic ward, the confused patient is most often suffering from *delirium*, which is an *acute onset* of altered consciousness that fluctuates over time. The symptoms include inattention, a failure of cognition (= knowledge of), or altered perception, including hallucinations. The end result is a misappreciation of date, time, or location in an individual who is often restless and may be verbally and physically aggressive.

Delirium is medically significant, and prevention of associated morbidity and mortality relies on careful clinical diagnosis.

PRECIPITATING FACTORS
Contributing causes of delirium are as follows:

1. *Old age:* The hospitalized elderly, who can become quickly confused after removal from their usual surroundings. Their situation may be worsened by sleep deprivation, deafness, visual impairment, and preexisting medical conditions.
2. *Preexisting dementia:* Patients with preexisting dementia are at high risk of developing acute onset of delirium.
3. *Head injury:* A period of confusion is common after or during the evolution of brain injury.
4. *Drugs:* Included here is recovery from general anesthesia and the side effects of opiate analgesia. Also, anticholinergics and benzodiazepines are common precipitants. Alcohol withdrawal and illicit drug abuse may also contribute.
5. *Pain:* Confusion may be associated with injury or result from the discomfort of visceral distension (e.g., urinary retention and constipation).
6. *Infection:* While chest infection is the classic postoperative cause of infection, other sources may be responsible (e.g., urinary tract and wound sites).

P. Wood et al., *Trauma and Orthopedic Surgery in Clinical Practice*,
DOI: 10.1007/978-1-84800-339-2_15, © Springer-Verlag London Limited 2009

7. *Hypoxia:* Pneumonia, fat embolism, pulmonary embolism, pulmonary contusion, and cardiac failure contribute to hypoxia.
8. *Metabolic:* Metabolic causes may be hyponatremia, or hypernatremia, hypoglycemia, renal impairment, and dehydration.
9. *Surgery:* Surgery is a cause, particularly after operation for a fractured neck of femur; often in association with one or more of the above factors.

THE ALCOHOLIC PATIENT

Alcohol-dependent patients will often attempt to conceal or minimize their drinking history. There is no typical alcoholic. Clues to the patient's actual intake may come from hospital notes concerning previous admissions, physical signs, and laboratory investigations (e.g., raised mean corpuscular volume [MCV] and liver function tests [LFTs]).

The first indication of trouble may be nonspecific anxiety and restlessness. This results from autonomic overactivity and may be associated with sweating, hypertension, and tachycardia. Severe cases may progress to convulsions or delirium tremens (DTs). DTs are a withdrawal syndrome characterized by confusion and bizarre visual hallucinations.

Your hospital may have an alcohol liaison team. If you suspect alcohol is a significant feature in the patient's history, then request an early referral for appropriate advice on managing potential withdrawal.

RISKS OF CONFUSION

Confused patients can become vocally and physically disruptive, thus presenting a hazard to themselves and others. The possibility of injury from falling when attempting to climb out of bed is a particular worry. Incontinence and difficulties over fluid balance and nutrition can make heavy demands on nursing staff. Consent for surgery is also a problem.

PRINCIPLES OF MANAGEMENT OF CONFUSION

The aim of confusion management is to find and correct any treatable cause from the list given in this chapter. This is easily stated, but in practice it is not always straightforward, particularly in elderly patients, for whom often no specific reason will be identified.

Throughout, the patient's care is heavily dependent on skilled nursing. On occasions, it may be necessary to sedate the patient for the safety of themselves and others. The aim is to do this with the minimal chemical insult possible. The practical danger is oversedation, and once hypnotics have been prescribed, a daily review of patient response versus dose is necessary.

Two drugs commonly employed are:

1. *Chlordiazepoxide:* This long-acting benzodiazepine is used in a stepwise reducing regime to treat alcohol withdrawal. Normally, 50–100 mg will be given by mouth, initially every 6 hours, with a stepwise reduction over several days. Alcoholic patients should also be prescribed parental B vitamins and oral thiamine (B_1) as nutritional supplements.
2. *Haloperidol:* This antipsychotic preparation is given in low doses to treat agitation and restlessness in the elderly, for which 0.5–1.5 mg orally once or twice a day will often be sufficient.

> The management of confusion demands clinical acumen and dedicated nursing.

FURTHER READING
See Chapter 8, The Patient With a Fractured Neck of Femur; Chapter 11, Infection and Immunocompromise; and Chapter 16, The Ill Patient and Medical Emergencies.

Chapter 16
The Ill Patient and Medical Emergencies

Most patients will undergo their orthopedic operation, recover uneventfully, and be discharged home. Some will unfortunately become sick. A number of problems may contribute, including:

1. Worsening of existing medical conditions: Elderly patients with chronic pulmonary or heart disease are at particular risk.
2. Infection: Wounds or systemic.
3. Embolism: Venous thrombosis or fat.
4. Compartment syndrome.
5. Confusion: Causes include items 1 to 3 (often associated with hypoxia), but hypoglycemia, dehydration, electrolyte disorders, and blood loss are also examples.
6. Idiosyncratic drug reactions, including anaphylaxis.
7. Problems with blood transfusion.

PRINCIPLES OF MANAGEMENT
The most important rule is that prevention is better than cure. Physiological derangement is best treated before disaster supervenes. The skill is to identify those patients who are demonstrating early warning signs and then to intervene before their condition changes from ill to critical.

Practical Management
When faced with an unwell patient, remember that common things occur commonly. A generic approach can be taken in managing these patients; be systematic and do the basics first.

History
Talk to the patient: Establish the recent history. What has happened and in what time frame? What are the patient's complaints? Is the

119

P. Wood et al., *Trauma and Orthopedic Surgery in Clinical Practice*, DOI: 10.1007/978-1-84800-339-2_16, © Springer-Verlag London Limited 2009

patient at risk for particular events such as pulmonary/fat embolism or sepsis?

Examination

Look at the patient:

Assess conscious level; if reduced establish that the patient is not diabetic (if so, quickly exclude hypoglycemia).

Is the reduced conscious level such that airway compromise and aspiration are threats? *Get help immediately (see the Very Ill Patient section).*

Look at the patient's color: Is the patient pale? Cyanosed? Flushed?

Check respiratory rate: Is it raised (infection, hemorrhage, hypoxia, anxiety, metabolic causes) or decreased (caused by central depression from drugs)?

Check pulse rate: Is it raised (infection, sepsis, hemorrhage, hypoxia, anxiety) or decreased (heart block, drug action)?

Check blood pressure: Is it low (sepsis, hemorrhage, primary cardiac event, anaphylaxis) or high (pain, essential hypertension)?

Check temperature: Is it raised? What does the surgical wound look like? Is it red? Swollen? Is it hot to touch? Is it smelly?

Check the drains: What is in them? Are they working as intended (chest drains in particular)?

Is the patient diabetic? Check the blood sugar and urine for ketones.

Are there infusions? What are they? Running as intended? Inspect fluid or drug delivery devices and infusion sites.

These key observations allow you to quickly identify likely problems and guide your subsequent management.

Look at the patient's records: Use the observations chart and any additional records to study the trends in temperature, pulse, blood pressure, respiratory rate, urine output, and oxygen saturation. If relevant, note the pain score and be clear regarding additional fluid losses from drains, sweat, diarrhea, and so on.

Also, review the patient's laboratory investigations, medication chart (in particular for drugs that could be directly influencing the patient's condition, e.g., steroids) and operation notes.

Investigate and Treat

Always try to interpret your examination findings in light of the patient's history and other evidence. Your response should include consideration of:

1. The need for urgent help: If so, get it immediately and while waiting initiate treatment as necessary (see The Very Ill Patient section and Table 16.1).
2. The need to make (or repeat) baseline investigations (e.g., chest X-ray [CXR], electrocardiogram [ECG], arterial blood gases, complete blood count (CBC), biochemistry profile (urea and electrolyte UEs), and investigations for sepsis.
3. The need to communicate the results of any investigations to your orthopedic seniors (always) and to other specialties as required.
4. A management plan for this patient: Further management of orthopedic complications will be as directed by your seniors, while medical problems will require referral to the appropriate specialty.

Ensure that you continue to see the "whole picture" and remain the coordinator between the various involved parties.

The Very Ill Patient

While we all have an intuitive grasp of what is meant by a *very ill patient*, a formal definition is not so easy, resting as it does on various imperfect physiological scoring systems. Here, we define it as a patient whose physiological status is such that the patient is in danger of reaching the potentially irretrievable position of respiratory or cardiorespiratory arrest. The early identification of such patients has received much study and is intimately linked to the work of the intensive care outreach team.

You are not expected to formally score patients, and what follows is a simple commonsense guide to assist you in identifying those patients who may be heading toward or already needing high-dependency or intensive care.

Some Facts Relevant in Physiological Deterioration

1. *Hypoxia kills*—and when this is an *acute* problem, it must be treated aggressively.
2. Learn to appreciate that a rising respiratory rate is often an early and sensitive index of developing problems. A persistent significant tachypnea (>30 breaths a minute) that is unrelated to anxiety or pain is a sure indicator of respiratory or circulatory pathology.
3. Remember that to some degree compensatory mechanisms will be working in the sick patient, and that patients who are already ill will succumb most easily to a failure of their reserves.

This observation extends to the results of blood gas analysis, which are the result of the primary disturbance and the body's physiological compensation. As a consequence, reasonable "numbers" may only be maintained at the expense of dangerous physical exhaustion.

In particular, do not be falsely reassured by satisfactory arterial saturations that are maintained with oxygen therapy. Arterial oxygen saturation may be normal in the presence of dangerous hypercapnia (carbon dioxide retention). In this situation, physical examination will reveal increasingly inadequate respiratory efforts because ventilation is failing. (Do not be distracted by the fact that oxygenation of patients with chronic obstructive pulmonary disease [COPD] can reduce their ventilatory drive; this is true, but the comment about oxygen saturation and hypercapnia can apply to *any* patient with respiratory failure).

4. Never be seduced by normotension in the face of persistent tachycardia; it will not stay this way indefinitely. Be aware of the secondary effects of hypotension (reduced conscious level, confusion, cardiac ischemia, reduced urine output).
5. Note that pyrexia and increased white cell count are not always matched. Be alert to the fact that the presence of one without the other can be a sinister sign of sepsis (see Chapter 11, Infection and Immunocompromise). Remember that the systemic effects of sepsis can produce hypotensive shock with devastating rapidity.

This Patient Is Suddenly Very Seriously Ill: What General Rules Should I Follow?

Immediately summon help, including the intensive care team (Figure 16.1)

In this situation, diagnosis and treatment are contemporaneous as the patient requires resuscitation. Your immediate priority is to identify life-threatening problems using ABC: *A* (airway), *B* (breathing), and *C* (circulation). Initiate treatment (Table 16.1) while help is en route.

If the patient is *unresponsive,* proceed as in Figure 16.2 (which assumes initially that you are the only medical practitioner, but appropriately qualified nurses are also in attendance).

If the patient is *conscious:*

Try not to leave the patient's side until help arrives.

Once help arrives, be ready to give a succinct relevant history of preceding events and thereafter undertake any tasks requested by the team leader.

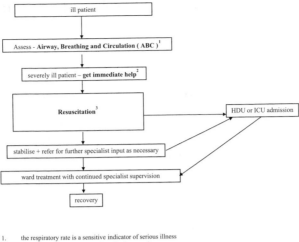

FIGURE 16.1. The postoperative patient. complications. HDU, high-dependency unit; ICU, intensive care unit.

While assistance is en route:

A: Give high-flow oxygen and attach an oximeter.

B: If the patient is in severe respiratory distress and has satisfactory blood pressure, sit the patient up.

C: Establish peripheral venous access if not already in place. Only start large-volume fluid infusion if you are sure that hypovolemia is present. If venous access is proving impossible, wait until help arrives.

Get the patient catheterized and ensure the collecting bag is a proper urometer. (If just catheterized and there is no urine at all, check—by performing a bladder washout—that the catheter tip is not blocked by the instillation jelly).

If the urine output is poor or nonexistent, do not reflexively administer a diuretic unless you are confident of a clinical diagnosis of left ventricular failure.

MEDICAL EMERGENCIES

More specific immediate actions to aid the management of some of the possible medical emergencies encountered in the perioperative period are outlined in Table 16.1.

1. Patient clearly very ill
request immediate help from intensive care team

2. Assess patient using ABC approach

A – open **airway** using jaw thrust or chin lift / head tilt
(if cervical collar present remove it and use jaw thrust only)

B – check for breathing for upto 10 seconds

C – check carotid pulse for upto 10 seconds

Breathing

normal – maintain airway + give O_2
exclude hypoglycaemia
Stay with patient until help arrives

wheezing – give O_2+/- nebulised beta adrenergic agonist
Stay with patient until help arrives

agonal breaths = cardiac arrest

Not breathing
Pulse present
call cardiac arrest team
Rescue breaths with pocket mask - 10/min
Check for pulse every 10 seconds

Not breathing
No Pulse
call cardiac arrest team + defibrillator
30 chest compressions followed by
2 rescue breaths - continue with 30:2 ratio until
defibrillator or arrest team arrives
- if defibrillator arrives first follow prompts if
AED model or otherwise shock if indicated

FIGURE 16.2.   The unresponsive patient: immediate actions. AED, automated external defibrillator.

TABLE 16.1. Medical Emergencies

Problem	Pathophysiology	Diagnosis	Treatment
Anaphylaxis	Type 1 hypersensitivity with histamine release; bronchospasm, hypotension	Symptoms usually occur immediately following exposure to precipitant; normally parenteral drug administration	Patient flat O_2 Adrenaline 0.5 mg im (= 0.5 mL of 1:1,000); repeat at 5 min if necessary Intravenous access + stat 1 L crystalloid Intravenous antihistamine (10–20 mg chlorphenamine) + 100 mg hydrocortisone iv Severe cases or laryngeal edema: Get immediate help
Angina	Cardiac ischemia worsened by hypoxia, hypotension, or anemia	Classic presternal discomfort (pressure or tightness) with radiation to left arm and neck May present as apparent indigestion or heartburn (also true for MI)	O_2 Sublingual nitrates; glyceryl trinitrate (400-μg spray in one or two metered doses or 300-μg tablet) Isosorbide dinitrate (1.25-mg spray in one to three metered doses or 10-mg tablet) Later check hemoglobin and correct if necessary If attacks prolonged or frequent, obtain ECG, take blood for myocardial troponins, and request urgent cardiology review

(Continued)

TABLE 16.1. Medical Emergencies

Problem	Pathophysiology	Diagnosis	Treatment
Acute coronary syndrome	Potential permanent injury to heart muscle from prolonged ischemia; precipitating factors same as for angina	Prolonged ischemic pain (>20 min) not relieved by nitrates; patient may be hypotensive ± experiencing arrhythmias 12-lead ECG may reveal ST changes or onset left bundle branch block (compare ECG with preop)	O_2 Stat 300 mg aspirin orally (chewed) Sublingual nitrates same as for angina Intravenous access + morphine analgesia, 1–2 mg intravenous boluses titrated to effect + antiemetic If available, attach patient to cardiac monitor (arrhythmias likely) Immediate cardiology + senior orthopedic consult as transfer to coronary care + thrombolysis may be indicated
Cardiac failure (pulmonary edema)	Exacerbation of chronic heart failure or secondary to pump failure in MI or from anemia	Anxiety + sweating Dyspnea; crepitations or wheeze on auscultation	Sit patient up O_2 Intravenous diuretic (40–80 mg frusemide) + intravenous morphine (1–2 mg; titrate to effect) Sublingual nitrates (not if hypotensive) Catheterize + urometer If history or ECG suggest possible acute cardiac event, then urgent cardiology opinion

Bronchospasm	Occurs as exacerbation of intrinsic asthma or COPD (often with associated chest infection) or during acute anaphylaxis	Tachypnea + tachycardia + increased effort of breathing + wheeze on auscultation (may be audible at bedside)	Ensure patient is sitting up; reassure (patients often very anxious) O_2 as carrier for nebulized salbutamol (2.5–5 mg) or terbutaline (5–10 mg) followed by 100 mg hydrocortisone iv Nebulized beta-2 agonists may need to be repeated, but if there is minimal response: 1. Get immediate help 2. Try nebulized ipratropium (500 µg) 3. *DO NOT* waste time attempting repeated arterial puncture if initially unsuccessful
Bradycardia	Depression of A-V conducting system; may be postinfarct	Clinical examination and 12-lead ECG Symptoms depend on effect on cardiac output • Syncope • Hypotension • Cardiac failure	Patient flat O_2 Intravenous atropine (500 µg) Repeat up to maximum of 3 mg Urgent cardiology opinion
Tachycardia	Pain, anxiety, cardiac arrhythmia (includes MI), pulmonary embolism, hemorrhage, sepsis (±pyrexia), hypercapnia, hypoxia, electrolyte imbalance	Clinical examination and 12-lead ECG Symptoms + signs depend on cause + effect on cardiac output; hypotension possible	If hypotensive, patient flat O_2 Correct according to presumed etiology If primary cardiac, urgent cardiology opinion

COPD, chronic obstructive pulmonary disease; ECG, electrocardiogram; MI, myocardial infarction.

Some Notes on Arterial Blood Gases

The usefulness of a blood gas sample may be increased if some basic rules are remembered:

1. Record whether the patient was breathing room air or, if receiving oxygen, the flow rate or inspired concentration if known.
2. The results need to be interpreted in light of both the patient's acute history and physical condition and any chronic illness. If the latter is present, make this clear when giving information over the phone.
3. With the exception of the partial pressure of oxygen, the values obtained from a peripheral venous sample will closely match those from arterial cannulation and therefore is itself valuable (particularly as the blood gas analyzer will also tell you the patients hemoglobin, sodium, potassium, and blood sugar).
4. If serial samples are available, the trends are often the important feature; record them in the notes by hand as the small flimsy results sheets produced by the blood gas machine are easily quickly lost.

Preparing for the Worst

Ask yourself:

Do I know the latest guidelines for in-hospital resuscitation? (Attendance at an advanced life support course may be a formal requirement during your first year of training.)

Do I know where the nearest defibrillator and resuscitation kit are located?

Have I been shown the defibrillator type and how it is checked and worked?

Would a quiet 5 minutes spent using a pocket face mask on a manikin have been useful?

In my hospital, who could I go to for informal advice and instruction in any of the above?

When the Worst Means Admission to Intensive Care

Try to accompany the patient with the intensive care unit (ICU) team. Watch their initial approach to treatment on arrival in ICU and ask questions. Learn from the experience and ask yourself whether there is anything that you could now do better if faced with the same situation again. Thereafter, maintain daily contact while the patient is in the ICU.

When the Worst Has Been Successfully Managed: Receiving Patients Discharged From the High-Dependency Unit or Intensive Care Unit

Never feel intimidated by patients discharged from the ICU or high-dependency unit. Until their condition has completely stabilized, they should remain the joint responsibility of yourself and the critical care team. Reception of such patients should occur early in the working day, and you need to make yourself available for a formal handover. Review such patient's progress on a daily basis and take advice as necessary over anything "unusual," such as a tracheostomy or functioning central venous lines.

Manage sick patients using the *ABC* approach. Tachypnea should never be ignored.

FURTHER READING
See Chapter 11, Infection and Immunocompromise; Chapter 13, Deep Venous Thrombosis and Pulmonary Embolism; Chapter 14, Fat Embolism and Chapter 17, problems with blood transfusion.

Chapter 17
Problems With Blood Transfusion

Blood transfusion is a common procedure; some 3 million units of red cells are given annually in the United Kingdom. When such large numbers are involved, it is inevitable that problems will occur. These may arise during the actual transfusion or during the pre- and posttransfusion periods. Difficulties can arise because of:

1. Nonhemolytic febrile reactions: These result from a donor white cell antigen/antibody reaction, the most common complication.
2. Fluid overload: This should be rare but may occur in the elderly.
3. Benign allergic reactions (rash, pruritis, urticaria) or true anaphylaxis (rare).
4. ABO blood group antigen incompatibility, an immune reaction from naturally occurring red cell antibodies causing intravascular hemolysis.
5. Transfusion-related lung injury (TRALI): Acute noncardiac pulmonary edema.
6. Infection from bacterial, parasitic, or viral contamination.
7. Posttransfusion purpura (PTP): Severe thrombocytopenia developing 5–10 days posttransfusion.

Nonhemolytic febrile reactions are usually self-limiting, but ABO incompatibility, TRALI, and bacterial contamination are all potentially lethal.

There are additional problems associated with massive transfusion, and some of the complications listed are more common during the administration of fresh frozen plasma and platelets. As these activities are rare events on an orthopedic ward, they will not be discussed further.

P. Wood et al., *Trauma and Orthopedic Surgery in Clinical Practice*, DOI: 10.1007/978-1-84800-339-2_17, © Springer-Verlag London Limited 2009

PRETRANSFUSION

The most likely problem pretransfusion is incorrect labeling of a blood sample taken for cross matching. As a consequence, it is likely that the *wrong blood is given to the wrong patient*—potentially causing a fatal transfusion reaction. The *correct procedure* for handling cross-match samples is discussed in the History, Physical Examination, and Clinical Investigations section of Chapter 4.

TRANSFUSION

Non hemolytic febrile responses occur 30 minutes or more after the transfusion has commenced. The temperature will rarely exceed 38.5°C, and there is usually no circulatory disturbance, although the patient may complain of feeling flushed.

True *hemolytic* reactions from ABO incompatibility occur soon after starting transfusion; the patient might experience chills, flushing, rigors, back or loin pain, and dyspnea accompanied by tachycardia, tachypnea, and hypotension. Urine output may decrease and darken in color; urinalysis will reveal hemoglobinuria.

TRALI usually presents during or within 6 hours of transfusion. The clinical signs and chest X-ray (CXR) will suggest a diagnosis of pulmonary edema, which in this case is due to lung injury.

Sepsis from bacterial contamination is rare but potentially rapidly fatal. The onset time and symptoms are the same as for ABO incompatibility, but there may be a high fever and diarrhea.

Anaphylaxis occurs most commonly in patients deficient for immunoglobulin A (IgA). It presents immediately after beginning a transfusion with signs of histamine release, including laryngeal edema, bronchospasm, and hypotension.

POSTTRANSFUSION

Both hemolytic and "transfusion lung" problems can be delayed. Hemolysis may manifest only after 1–3 weeks as an unexpectedly low posttransfusion hemoglobin or jaundice. PTP will require detailed hematological investigation; heparin-induced thrombocytopenia is a differential diagnosis in those patients receiving thromboprophylaxis.

RESPONDING TO A TRANSFUSION PROBLEM

The critical distinction of a transfusion problem is between simple nonhemolytic reactions and hemolysis from ABO-incompatible blood. If the patient is mildly febrile but otherwise well, stop the transfusion and check that the patient's identity band details correspond to that of the unit being transfused (Figure 17.1). Thereafter, continue but decrease the rate of transfusion and give paracetamol for the temperature. Following this, the patient must be frequently reassessed until the transfusion is completed.

However, if there are obvious cardiorespiratory changes in a patient who is clearly unwell *or* if you are uncertain, then:

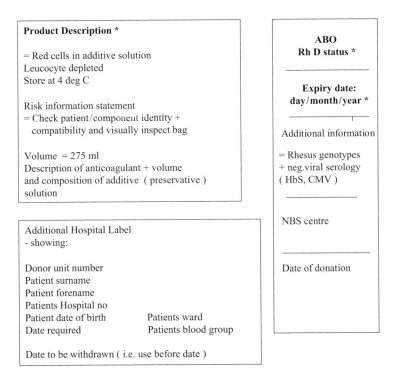

Donor unit number *

Product Description *

= Red cells in additive solution
Leucocyte depleted
Store at 4 deg C

Risk information statement
= Check patient/component identity +
   compatibility and visually inspect bag

Volume = 275 ml
Description of anticoagulant + volume
and composition of additive (preservative)
solution

**ABO
Rh D status ***

─────────────────

**Expiry date:
day/month/year ***

─────────────────

Additional information

= Rhesus genotypes
+ neg.viral serology
(HbS, CMV)

─────────────────

NBS centre

─────────────────

Date of donation

Additional Hospital Label
- showing:

Donor unit number
Patient surname
Patient forename
Patients Hospital no
Patient date of birth   Patients ward
Date required   Patients blood group

Date to be withdrawn (i.e. use before date)

Note - Figure is based on four quadrant model in which all blocks marked *
have a unique printed bar code which is designed to minimise error at every
stage from the point of donation to eventual transfusion

FIGURE 17.1. What are you prescribing? Information displayed on the front of a unit of packed red cells (drawn from an actual unit given during surgery).

Stop the transfusion and assess the patient using the *ABC* approach.

If the patient is very sick get help from the intensive care team. Thereafter, be prepared to help investigate the donated blood in conjunction with the transfusion laboratory (this is a statutory requirement). Do the following:

1. Give supplemental oxygen.
2. Examine the respiratory and cardiovascular system:

   If the patient is hypotensive but normovolemic, then give intravenous saline as renal perfusion must be maintained if there is any possibility of hemolysis.

   If the patient is elderly, look for signs of fluid overload. If there is obvious cardiac failure, administer an intravenous diuretic.
3. Anaphylaxis must be treated with adrenaline (see Chapter 16, The Ill Patient and Medical Emergencies).
4. Catheterize the patient and consider the need for a portable CXR.
5. Remember if ABO incompatibility has occurred because of mistaken identity, then it is possible that another patient is danger. Inform the blood bank and follow their instructions. They will want the unit bags in question returned plus your paper copy of the transfusion record and venous samples from the patient, which in any case should include a full blood count, repeat grouping, coagulation screen, and blood cultures.
6. While writing up the patient's notes, record the identity numbers of the questionable units in case the separate transfusion records should get lost.

> The single biggest misadventure from blood transfusion is logistical error pretransfusion.

FURTHER READING

See the History, Physical Examination, and Clinical Investigations section in Chapter 4; Chapter 5, Intravenous Fluids and Electrolytes; and Chapter 16, The Ill Patient and Medical Emergencies.

Section 5

Problems and Complications:
The Doctor

Chapter 18
Medical Errors

BACKGROUND

Complications are an integral part of anesthesia and surgery. Even with the best care, some patients will suffer complications and an adverse outcome; examples in orthopedics are deep venous thrombosis (DVT), pulmonary embolism (PE), and wound infection. These and other complications are discussed in the relevant chapters.

The aim is to be alert to the possibility of these problems and ideally recognize them early. This will mean effective treatment can be better given and the patient's outcome improved.

However, much of what "goes wrong" is *avoidable*. It is estimated that up to 10% of hospital inpatients suffer a medical mishap, of which some 50% were preventable. This last figure is high because many of these errors result from basic slips.

We all make mistakes. Most are minor and self-limiting; others are not. The current medical landscape includes a patient population whose tolerance for medical error is not what it was.

CAUSES OF MEDICAL ERROR AND AVOIDING THEM

We confine our comments here to the routine everyday tasks that have the potential to catch you out. Of these, "written" errors are the greatest concern. The list that follows is particularly relevant for those not working with electronic prescribing systems. If such a facility is used in your hospital, it is essential that you are fully educated in its usage.

1. Write legibly at all times. The old jokes about doctors' handwriting are no longer funny.
2. When prescribing drugs, print the name and use generic names only. When checking the dose of a drug, use the current edition of the *British National Formulary* (BNF), or equivalent.

P. Wood et al., *Trauma and Orthopedic Surgery in Clinical Practice*,
DOI: 10.1007/978-1-84800-339-2_18, © Springer-Verlag London Limited 2009

3. Be careful in distinguishing between milligrams and micrograms and in the use of decimal points.
4. Write insulin doses as units, not as U, which may look like a zero.
5. If the prescription involves any "calculating," particularly with respect to infusions, check your math with a colleague.
6. If your prescription is "challenged" by nursing or pharmacy staff, review it as a priority.
7. Patient identity: Are you giving the correct treatment to the right patient? Be very aware when the ward contains more than one patient with the same surname. Be certain of identity when matching and labeling patient samples with clinical request forms. Do not become distracted by nonurgent matters during such tasks. Remember the biggest problem in blood transfusion misadventure is logistical.
8. Operating lists: Again, legible writing is the key. Print and do not abbreviate. Check that limbs have been marked correctly.
9. X-rays are utilized everywhere on an orthopedic ward. When planning a patient's care, check that the films on the viewing screen are indeed those of the patient in question, and that it is the correct limb or area, properly oriented on the screen.
10. Always respond in a timely and professional manner to nurses' requests to review either a patient's clinical condition or their prescriptions.

WHAT TO DO IF YOU HAVE MADE A MISTAKE

If the patient has or is likely to come to harm if you have made a mistake, the following approach is suggested:

1. Inform your consultant immediately so actions can be initiated to limit or reverse any actual damage.
2. Insert a full description of events in the patient's notes.
3. Apologize to the patient and offer a full explanation of what has gone wrong. The medical-legal experts tell us that this action is the single most important factor in reducing the chances that the patient will subsequently seek legal address. Note that this action does not equate to an admission of liability.
4. Fill in a critical incident form.
5. Be prepared for a postincident debriefing by your consultant and possibly a clinical risk manager. The latter may require a written statement from you. It is always wise to draft such a statement while events are fresh in your mind.
6. Have a low threshold for discussing any aspect of the problem with your medical indemnity organization; in particular, you

may well be advised to copy any prepared statements to them. In the U.K. health service, you are protected by your employers from the financial consequences of clinical mishap, but your defense organization can also be a source of help and clinical advice.

7. Do not at any stage lie to yourself or others.

To err is human. It is most unlikely that you are the only person ever to have committed this particular sin.

Learn from it and move on. If you find the event so upsetting that it begins to seriously disrupt your daily activities, do not delay in informing your consultant or occupational health advisor, who should ensure that you receive professional help.

> Patients appreciate the truth. Apology and admission of guilt are not necessarily equivalent.

FURTHER READING
See Chapter 4, Preparing Patients for Operation, Parts I and II; the entire Section 4, Problems and Complications: The Patient.

Section 6
When Treatment Stops

Chapter 19
Do Not Resuscitate Orders, Death Certification, and the Coroner

WHEN FURTHER TREATMENT IS THOUGHT INAPPROPRIATE

One of the most important areas of medicine is knowing when not to initiate additional treatment or when to actively withdraw parts of it. Such decisions are difficult even when years of experience are applied to the problem. The public is well aware of this, and respecting patients' and families' wishes can occasionally invite ethical and legal conflict.

On a general orthopedic ward, such cases are rare but occasionally occur, for instance, when caring for infirm patients with a fractured neck of femur. Your role is to be aware of the overall treatment plan and refer to your seniors any issues, raised by the patient or the patient's family, that appear to conflict with this plan.

DO NOT RESUSCITATE ORDERS

Do not resuscitate (DNR) orders are not unusual. They are directives either prepared in advance by the patient or arising de novo after discussion with the patient (and ideally the patient's family or caregivers) by senior medical and nursing staff.

The orders acknowledge that cardiopulmonary resuscitation in terminally ill patients is often inappropriate. They should be made solely on the basis of the patient's current morbidity and likely prognosis.

The DNR orders should be recorded on designated forms and be kept prominent in the patient's notes. It is usual practice to review the statement at regular intervals, which may be as frequent as every 24 hours.

It is essential that you are aware for which, if any, of your patients such documentation exists.

P. Wood et al., *Trauma and Orthopedic Surgery in Clinical Practice*,
DOI: 10.1007/978-1-84800-339-2_19, © Springer-Verlag London Limited 2009

CERTIFICATION OF DEATH

A medical certificate of cause of death should only be issued when you are satisfied regarding the cause. Before signing, it is necessary in the United Kingdom to observe the 14-day rule, which is you must have attended the patient some time in the 14 days before death (28 days in Northern Ireland) or else seen the patient after death.

If the medical team is not clear regarding the cause of death, then no certificate is issued until the case has been discussed with the coroner (see the Reporting to the Coroner section).

CREMATION CERTIFICATES

You may be asked to sign the first part (known helpfully as Form B) of a cremation certificate. To do this, you must see and externally examine the body in the presence of a more senior colleague (one who has been qualified for 5 or more years).

POSTMORTEMS

Hospital postmortems are becoming increasingly rare. Although any grade of doctor can request one from the next of kin, it is very likely that, if thought desirable, this task would be undertaken by the most senior doctor treating the patient. Such requests must obviously be handled with great sensitivity. Some relatives will want time to "think about it," following which it is possible that a family member might approach you with specific questions about what exactly happens at autopsy, for instance, with respect to retention of organs or tissue for teaching and research purposes. A good form of prior preparation is to familiarize yourself with your hospital's postmortem request form, which in the United Kingdom is likely to be based on a model supplied by the Human Tissue Authority (HTA). The consent form is subdivided so that specific aspects of the postmortem such as tissue or organ retention can receive separate and individualized consent as necessary. (A link to the HTA's new code of practice document on postmortem examination is included in our Bibliography).

REPORTING TO THE CORONER

In the United Kingdom, the following circumstances must be reported to the coroner or the coroner's deputizing officer (a police officer):

1. All deaths for which the medical staff are uncertain regarding the actual cause of death.
2. All deaths occurring within 24 hours of admission to the hospital.

3. Death following an operation or medical procedure or if there was no recovery from anesthetic.
4. Death following an accident.
5. Death related to industrial disease.
6. If there is uncertainty over the circumstances leading to death or there was a violent or unnatural death.

If in doubt, talk to the coroner's office. Following discussion with you, they will either direct you to sign a death certificate or they will order a coroner's postmortem (this cannot be refused by next of kin), which may or may not become part of a coroner's inquest.

End-of-life issues must be handled with due sensitivity while also observing the laws of the land.

Bibliography and Further Reading

We have provided external references as a supplement because several include material that is relevant to one or more sections of the book. The emphasis in our selection has been to provide sources that are committed to remaining updated.

YOUR WORK PLACE

Intranet/trainees handbook/induction package: Your trust will have "in-house" protocols for many of the situations discussed in this book; if so, follow them.

WEB SITES

British National Formulary: www.BNF.org. Electronic version of the *British National Formulary* (see Books section).Department of Health: www.dh.gov.uk/. It is not easy to navigate around this monster but using the search facility will provide links to policy and guidance for most clinical situations.

British Thoracic Society: www.brit-thoracic.org.uk/. Key source for management of pulmonary embolism.

General Medical Council: www.gmc-uk.org/. The section "Guidance for Doctors" leads to Consent: patients and doctors making decision together (2008), which deals comprehensively with issues of consent.

Health Protection Agency: www.hpa.org.uk/. Independent body that reports and advises on hospital acquired infections.

Human Tissue Authority: www.hta.gov.uk. Has a guidance section that includes a code of practice on postmortem examination.

National Institute for Clinical Excellence: www.nice.org.uk/. Has an index of published guidelines, including extensive material on preoperative investigations.

National Patient Safety Agency: www.npsa.nhs.uk. Has a patient incident reporting scheme through which you can report (anonymously if desired) actual or "near-miss" incidents.

Royal College of Surgeons of England: www.rcseng.ac.uk. Contains a checklist for correct site surgery.

Scottish Intercollegiate Guidelines: www.sign.ac.uk/. Has numbered guideline publications on many perioperative issues.

U.K. blood transfusion and tissue transfusion services: www.transfusion guide/.org.uk. Best practice advice on blood transfusion.

U.K. Committee for Standards in Haematology: www.bcshguidelines.com. Also publishes guidelines on transfusion issues.

U.K. Resuscitation Council: www.resus.org.uk/. Important because changes to the resuscitation guidelines first appear here.

U.K. Royal College of Radiologists: www.rcr.ac.uk. Has a publication section that includes indications for preoperative chest X-rays: "Making the Best Use of Clinical Radiology Services" (6th ed., 2007).

JOURNALS AND SUPPLEMENTS

British Medical Journal. Editorials and clinical reviews often provide concise résumés of current clinical practice or thinking. In addition, the journal publishes a series of practical clinical guides under the blanket title "ABC of ...." These are designed with medical students and junior clinicians in mind, and several (e.g., blood transfusion) are relevant to the orthopedic ward.

BOOKS

British National Formulary. Your pharmacological and prescribing bible. Also available electronically at www.BNF.org. Published by the British Medical Association and the Royal Pharmaceutical Society of Great Britain. The current edition is number 55 (March 2008).

Index

A

American society of
anesthesiologists (ASA)
score, 36
Analgesia, 21
pain treating methods
control factors and
assessment, 65–66
local anesthetics, 67–68
opiates and analgesics, 67
3 P's treatments, 66
practical analgesic issues
respiratory depression, 68
spinal cord compression, 69
Anaphylaxis, 125, 133–134
Anesthesia, 33
Anticoagulant drugs and spinal/
epidural anesthesia dosing, 50
Arterial blood gases, 121, 128
Asthma, 33

B

Bacteremia, 95–96, 99–101
Biguanide, 43. *See also* Diabetes
Blood transfusion
actual, 133
blood gas samples, 128
elective surgery
and blood transfusion
laboratory, 36–37
fatal transfusion reaction, cause
of, 132
maximum surgical blood order
schedule (MSBOS), 37
non hemolytic febrile responses,
133
pre and post transfusion,
132–133

problems, 131
intravenous treatments, 134
respondance, 133–134
service and donations, 60
British national formulary
(BNF), 137

C

Cardiac failure, 31
Chlordiazepoxide and confusion
management, 117
Chronic obstructive pulmonary
disease (COPD), 32, 95, 122
Chronic respiratory disease, 79
Clostridium difficile infection,
98–100
Compartment syndrome in trauma
patients
cause of, 103
compartment pressure
measurement, 105–106
fractures and, 103
management pathway for, 105
standard fracture care, 104
symptoms and prevention, 104
treatment, 106–107
Computerized tomographic (CT)
imaging, 114
computerized tomographic
pulmonary angiography
(CPTA), 111
venography, 109
Coroner and report of death,
144–145
C-Reactive protein (CRP)
level, 96
Cremation certificate, 144
Critical care outreach team, 21

D
Death certification, 144
Deep venous thrombosis (DVT),
47, 137
    diagnosis, 109
    treatment of, 110
Delirium tremens (DTs), 115–116
Diabetes
    glycemic control, 45
    insulin-dependent diabetes
        mellitus (IDDM), 43
    non-insulin-dependent diabetes
        mellitus (NIDDM), 43
    patient preoperative protocol, 45
    and surgery, 43–44
Dipyridamole, 47
Do not resuscitate (DNR) orders, 143

E
Electrocardiogram (ECG), 31, 83,
    88, 110, 114, 121
Erythrocyte sedimentation rate
    (ESR), 96, 114

F
Fat embolism
    associations, 113
    diagnosis confirmation, 114
    treatment, 114
Fluid management
    practical observations, 60, 63
Fractured neck of femur (NOF),
    patient with, 79
    dynamic hip screw (DHS), 82
    management
        pathway for, 84
        principles of, 81
    operating theater preparation
        for, 83
    surgical classification
        intracapsular femoral neck
            fractures, 79–81
        subtrochanteric fractures, 81
        trochanteric fractures and basal
            femoral neck fractures, 81

G
Glomerular filtration rate (GFR), 83

H
Haloperidol and confusion
    management, 117
Health care-associated infections
    (HCAIs), 98
Health protection agency
    (HPA), 99
Heart disease, patients preparation
    for operation
    blood pressure measurements, 32
    pacemaker functions, 32
Hemophilia
    orthopedic presentation, 89–90
    postoperative care
        blood salvage techniques, 90
        HIV immunosuppression, 91
    preoperative preparation
        factor levels, 90
        prophylactic treatment, 89
Heparin, 47
    and deep venous thrombosis, 110
High-dependency unit (HDU), 54
Human tissue authority
    (HTA), 144
Hypertonic saline dextran (HSD), 59
Hypoglycemia, 44

I
Ill patient and medical
        emergencies, 119–129
    management principles
        history and examination in,
            119–120
        investigation and treatment,
            120–121
        practical, 119–121
        very ill patient, 121–123
    postoperative patient
        complications, 123
    serious case and, 122–123
    unresponsive patient, 124
Infection and immunocompromise
    history and examination, 96
    infection-sepsis pathway, 97
    laboratory and radiological
        investigation, 96
    management principles
        rules for, 99, 101

orthopedic patients and hospital
  infections, 95–96
postoperative
  health care-associated
    infection, 98
  iatrogenic, 99
  methicillin-resistant
    Staphylococcus aureus
    and *Clostridium difficile*
    infections, 99–100
  sepsis, 96–98
  risks, 101
In-hospital resuscitation, 128
Intensive care unit (ICU), 21, 54
  admission in, 128
  discharged patients, 129
International normalized ratio
  (INR), 110
Intravenous fluids and electrolytes
  fluid characteristics, 57
    artificial colloids, 58–59
    blood and blood products, 60
    hypertonic crystalloids, 59–60
    isotonic crystalloids, 58
  fluid management, 60, 63
  sodium and potassium problems,
    61–62 (*See also* Orthopedic
    patients)
Ischemic heart disease, 87–88

L
Latex allergy, 35
  natural rubber latex (NRL), 35
  routine clinical investigations, 35
Liver diseases, 89
  liver function tests (LFTs), 116
Low molecular weight heparins
  (LMWHs), 110

M
Magnetic resonance imaging (MRI)
  scan, 51
Mean corpuscular volume
  (MCV), 116
Medical errors
  approach after, 138–139
  causes and avoidance, 137–138
  written, 137–138

Medication
  chronic medical conditions, 37
  fasting, 38–41
  nothing-by-mouth policy, 42
  principles and practical
    considerations, 37–38
Methicillin-Resistant
    Staphylococcus aureus
    (MRSA) infections, 98–100
Morphine, 66–67

N
National Institute for Clinical
    Excellence (NICE)
    protocols, 36
Neck of femur (NOF), 32
Neurology
  epidural *in’situ* and cord
    compression, 51
  and sickle cell disease patients
    preparation, 33
Nonsteroidal anti-inflammatory
    drugs (NSAIDs), 67, 83

O
Orthopedic patients
  alcoholic, 116
  confused patient
    drugs for, 117
    management principles, 116–117
    risks of, 116
  imaging modalities, 17–19
  operation
    postoperative management
      of, 71–75
    problems after, 119
  orthopedic terms, 10–15
  perioperative drugs, 39–41
  and procedures, 3
    orthopedic ward, 4–9
  very ill patient
    physiological deterioration,
      121–122
  ward round
    description and types of, 24–25
    patient's medical care, 23
  ward team
    acute pain control and, 21

Orthopedic patients preparation
for operation
blood transfusion laboratory,
36–37
consent and identification
anesthesia, 53–54
elective surgery for, 52
operating list, 54–55
purpose-designed consent
forms, 53
diabetic patient, 43–46
fasting periods, 38, 42
medical, 29, 31
with neurology and an epidural
in situ, 51
problems during history and
physical examination
drugs on admission, 34, 37
heart diseases, 31–32
latex allergy, 35
neurological deficits, 33
patients with pacemaker, 32
pregnancy, 34
previous anesthesia,
suxamethonium apnea, 35
renal disease, 33
respiratory disease, 32–33
sickle cell disease, 34
routine clinical investigations,
35–36
spinal cord compression, 51
thromboembolic complications,
46–50

P
Patient-controlled analgesia
(PCA), 66
Physiotherapist role in
postoperative progress, 21
Postmortems, 144
Postoperative nausea and vomiting
(PONV), 68–69
Posttransfusion purpura (PTP),
131, 133
Pregnancy patients preparation
anesthesia, 34
Preoperative assessment clinic,
29, 31

Pulmonary embolism (PE), 109, 137
key features of, 111
sick patient and, 112
treatment of, 112

R
Renal disease
patients preparation for
operation
predialysis renal impairment,
33
Respiratory disease
patients preparation for
operation
asthmatic patients, 33
nebulizer therapy and, 33
Rheumatoid arthritis
postoperative care and infections
gastrointestinal symptoms, 88
preoperative dehydration, 88
preparation for surgery, 87

S
Sepsis, 95–96, 133
ABC approach, 98
infection pathway, 97
septic shock, 95
Spinal cord compression
symptoms and signs of, 51
Sulfonylurea, 43
Surgery
identification of
correct patient for correct
operation, 54
pathway for, 30
reasonable guidelines for
elective, 52
and surgical diabetic ladder, 44
Systemic inflammatory response
syndrome (SIRS), 95, 97

T
Thromboprophylaxis
activated partial thromboplastin
time (APPT), 110
anticoagulant drugs dosing of, 50
low molecular weight heparin
(LMWH), 47

patient history, factors and
    operative procedures, 46–47
techniques and drugs used for, 47
Transfusion-related lung injury
    (TRALI), 131, 133
Trauma, 60, 68, 79, 101, 103
  acute trauma, 42

V
Valvular heart disease, 32, 48
Volkmann's ischemic
    contracture, 103

W
Warfarin, 32, 47–49

Printed in the United States